Nurturing
Mind, Body, and Soul

Nurturing
Mind, Body, and Soul

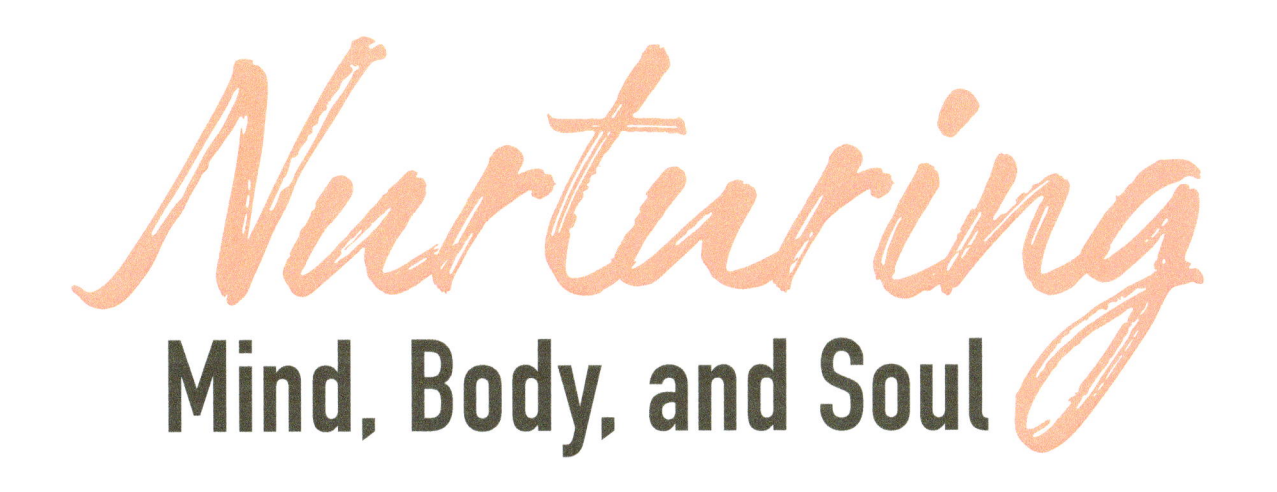

**Demystifying the Journey
with Christine Crawford**

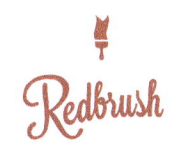

Redbrush

Copyright © 2024 by Christine Crawford

All rights reserved. No part of this book may be reproduced, scanned, or distributed in any printed or electronic form without direct permission from the author or publisher.

Cover Photography:
Lisa Leanne Photography

Styling/Design/Florals:
Glenna Joy Flowers & Arbor Love Art

Calligraphy:
Lazy Creative Designs

First Edition: May 2024
Printed in the United States of America

ISBN: 979-8-9893590-0-4 (printed edition)
        979-8-9893590-1-1 (eBook edition)

Printed by

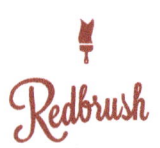

Redbrush

Foreword

I was deeply touched when Christine Crawford asked me to write the foreword to her book, 'Nurturing Mind, Body, and Soul'. Christine was an amazing, intuitive student at HMI College of Hypnotherapy in Tarzana, Ca. I had the privilege of having her in my classes Medical Hypnosis, Child Hypnosis, and Ethics and Law. She impressed me by understanding that the true key to positive change comes from Self Compassion, Mindfulness, and PRACTICE! Christine doesn't just talk the talk, she walks the walk. I got to know Christine during our many walks on the beach in beautiful Southern California, while we discussed daily practices to have a superior quality of life and be present in the present moment. We also discussed how to make a goal into a plan, and then execute that plan beginning, middle and end to complete what we had started. It's no surprise that one of the goals we talked about is WRITING AND PUBLISHING A BOOK on creating a better, healthier, and happier life that everyone could access and apply.

'Nurturing Mind, Body, and Soul' is an easy and practical formula that everyone can understand. It is filled with daily practices that nurture the mind, body, and soul. Filled with excellent research, this book is based not only on personal experience, but also solid scientific evidence. Christine effortlessly combines the best of her own education, experience, and expertise, with personal stories and research from scientific and psychological communities.

I teach at an International Vocational College, have a private practice on Zoom and in person, have three children, and a retired husband enjoying my company at home. Like many of us, I don't have time for formal meditation every day. Instead, I follow Christine's Walking Mindfulness and Eating Mindfulness, which fit perfectly into even my busiest days. I'm able to SAVOR the moment despite a rigorous, demanding schedule. The secret that makes this book superior to other "Self-Help Books," is its ease of use. When you pick just one thing to do every day, you can see the difference in your life in days, not weeks, months or years. And you, like me, can choose a different exercise every day if you enjoy variety as much as I.

Christine graduated HMI College in 2022. She has a keen understanding of how the subconscious mind influences our actions. Logic, reason, and will power (those things never there when you need them) are only a fraction of the mind. The Sub Conscious wants to repeat familiar patterns, even if they are against self care. Because of her training in Hypnotherapy, Ms. Crawford gives us small, easy but powerful changes that make all the difference. As they say in AA, "It Works if you Work it". With 'Nurturing Mind, Body, and Soul', you get a program that indeed "works when you work it". The difference is that it is so accessible, it becomes easy, automatic, and amazingly effective for long-term superior positive change.

Lisa R. Machenberg
Instructor HMI College of Hypnotherapy
Host of Amazing Mind and Hypnosis Today

Preface

Man...He sacrifices his health in order to make money. Then he sacrifices money to recuperate his health. And then he is so anxious about the future that he does not enjoy the present; the result being that he does not live in the present or the future; he lives as if he is never going to die, and then dies having never really lived.
—***The 14th Dalai Lama***

Life is for the living, and by living, I don't mean getting by. Life is for experiencing the great and small, appreciating everyday moments, and doing what interests us—living out our dreams.

So, if this is true, why aren't we living our lives to the fullest? I meet so many people who are alive yet dead. They're not thriving, and they're not flourishing. They are stuck in a rut, lethargic, or filled with pain and anxiety.

Unfortunately, in this stressful environment, we risk not experiencing our lives. We struggle with daily activities of meeting deadlines and paying bills. We foster unhealthy relationships with ourselves lacking in love, compassion, and acceptance. We don't think about our connection with the spiritual world or our ability to experience joy. We simply do not have time.

Twenty years ago, I was a wife and new mother in the beautiful idyllic town of Westlake Village, California. There were multitudes of families with young children scattered around my neighborhood. The weather was always good. I met many new mothers at the local mom's club, and we met regularly. While our kids would play, we would discuss motherhood and life in Westlake Village. My husband worked as a partner in a law firm in downtown Los Angeles. He would play golf and fish in the local lake on the weekends. I had experienced several miscarriages, but now I had my angel, my boy. Life couldn't have been more perfect, or so it would seem.

Unfortunately, this state of bliss slowly began to slip away. My son had what doctors called colic from birth until three months of age, and as such, I barely got three hours of sleep a day. My relationship with my husband of thirteen years deteriorated. I spent all my energy trying to appease my child, in part by finding foods that made him happy. With little time and energy left to take care of myself, I was left finishing his goldfish crackers or other kid food. I developed digestive issues. I gained ten pounds and wasn't exercising.

I started drinking alcohol more regularly—at mom's night out and on many other occasions. I found that a glass of wine—or several—in the evening helped me forget my troubles, which caused me to have brain fog and difficulty sleeping at night. I struggled daily through a wine-induced stupor, waking up groggy and irritable with a headache and drained of energy. "What was that movie we watched last night?" I couldn't remember the ending. As I struggled to make the coffee to relieve my headache, I realized I had to clean the house. *Ugh, my least favorite task.*

Angry at my husband and son for being slobs, I would have an ugly scowl. I would feel unhealthy and needed to eat, but I had to feed my son Mak first. I would see my husband off to work, shower, and get dressed. Having gained some weight, I would look in the mirror and not like my appearance. Too many wrinkles, chubby face. "I should exercise, but I don't have time for that." Running late and still needing to eat, I would take a big spoonful of peanut butter and head out the door. I would take Mak to a playdate and have a nice time chatting with the other moms. They would break out the wine, and I would be thrilled to partake. I needed it to "take the edge off." Everyone would bring something to eat. We would have lunch, usually full of cheese and carbs.

When we got home, I would be so tired I had to lie down with Mak as he napped. I'd wake up an hour later feeling groggy and awful, my stomach bloated and crampy. I would want to go back to sleep, but Mak would wake up soon. I would prepare his afternoon snack and have my late afternoon snack, something I would throw in the microwave. Mak and I would play with Legos until Dad got home from work, and we would make dinner. Dinner was our most healthful meal, as my husband cooked. We usually had beef or pork with pasta or rice and a glass of wine. We had vegetables occasionally. Sometimes we would have a good time preparing our dinner, but more often than I liked, we would argue about something. After dinner, I would put Mak and myself to bed. The following day, Mak would wake up bright and early, crying, and I would wake up groggy with my half-finished glass of wine on my bedside table. Put this on repeat, day after day, for years.

Desperate for a change, I stumbled across some great information via articles from an old high school friend. They were about holistic health and connecting to the soul. They talked about becoming the person we truly want to be. I was enthralled.

This new information struck a chord in my heart and brought a strong urge in me, a need for change. So I started studying nutrition and health. I experimented with food, how it made me feel and how it affected my body regarding my food sensitivity issues. Food has always been a focal point in my life. Before my son was born, I loved cooking and food-related experiences. I read a lot about Italy's food culture and decided to expand my knowledge. The food culture there is delicious, healthy, and exciting. My husband assured me my son would be okay with him while I was away, so I booked my flight.

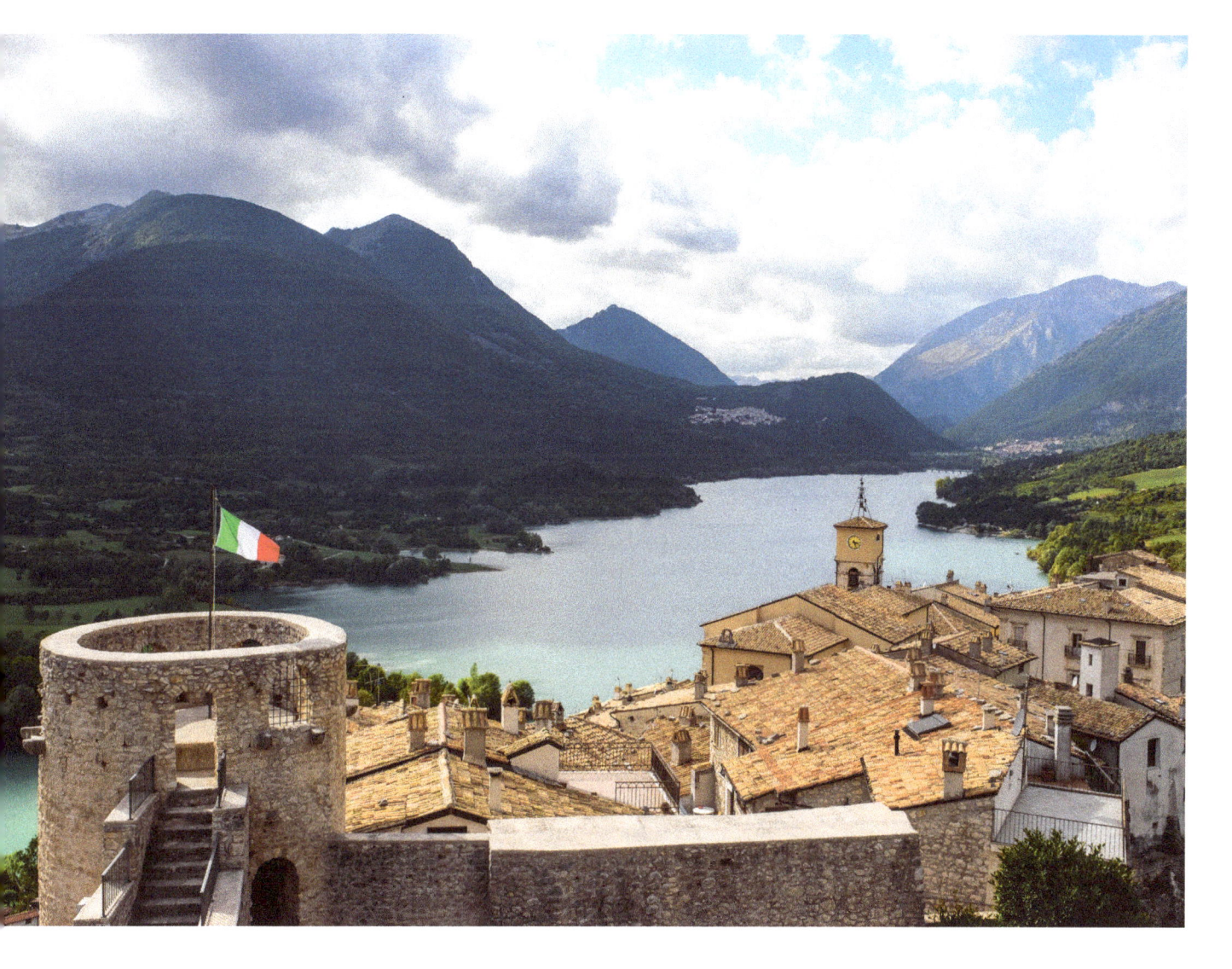

During my time in Italy, I enjoyed taking in new sights, smells, sounds, and tastes. I immersed myself fully in the moment, and it changed my perspective.

A few of my encounters stood out and had a lasting effect. I enjoyed Rome and other tourist areas, but I noticed the food tasted like something I would get in any big city like New York City, Paris, or London. Then I happened upon the *agriturismos* in the countryside, which was a different story altogether. An agriturismo is like a bed and breakfast at a small farm or farmhouse resort. The Italian government created agriturismos to save rural architecture and Italy's small farms. As such, farmers who convert part of their property into an agriturismo get financial help from the government. One of the things that I admire about Italian culture is that they put great value on small-scale, family-run production of foods such as olives, wine, and cheese, and this was the perfect embodiment of those values.

I had a room at the farm, and the package included meals. So when I joined the communal dining table, I was surprised to experience some of the most amazing meals of my life. Because they raised the chickens, grew the vegetables, handmade the pasta, and milked the goats for cheese, the food was incomparable and some of the best I've had.

One particular night in Abruzzo was unforgettable. I was at a working farm that produces its own wine, olive oil, jam, and cheese. It was an excellent spot in the middle of vineyards and olive trees, with fabulous views of the Adriatic and surrounding countryside. They had just brought in freshly picked truffles, so we were in for a treat for dinner. The refreshing mountain and sea air, combined with the newly shaved truffles, made me feel like I was in the best dream I'd ever had.

The homemade pasta and cream sauce, complemented by the freshly shaved truffles, is something I will always remember. The difference between the truffle pasta I had in Rome a few days before and this was unbelievable. The truffles had a mellower, rounded, exquisite flavor. The slightly al dente, homemade tagliatelle pasta was the perfect match. The cream sauce and cheese were from freshly milked goats, and they used herbs just picked from their garden. I had never experienced fresh and delicious ingredients pulled together by centuries-old Italian recipes.

When I returned to Los Angeles, I dedicated myself to cooking natural, unprocessed foods with the freshest ingredients possible. I found most of what I sought at farmer's markets, which offer locally grown, seasonal, and organic options.

At age forty-five, I had a hunger, a mission, a destiny—something I hadn't had in a long time—so I decided to attend nutrition school. I studied and eventually became a board-certified holistic health expert. I specialized in art and music therapy, along with hypnotherapy. I started a *real* food blog (www.realyummieswithchris.com) and regularly contributed to a magazine in my area with recipes, photos, and articles on well-being. "Finding myself" in this manner changed my life. My son was and still is the most important thing in my life, but I couldn't take care of my son until I took care of myself first. My relationship with my husband improved dramatically. I became a better and more attentive mother to my son, and I was better to myself.

Today, a Saturday, I woke up, made my coffee, and had oatmeal with apples, blueberries, and walnuts. I always have a glass of water with me throughout the day. I did some painting in my studio with classical music playing, and then I had lunch. I had an omelet with wild mushrooms, fresh chives, thyme, tarragon, and turmeric. Then I went to our local orphanage and decorated the gym for a Halloween party for the kids there. Afterward, I returned home to spend time with my family. I had a snack of persimmons and pistachios. I walked the dogs. It was a gorgeous autumn day, and I thoroughly enjoyed the sights, smells, and sounds every step of the way. At home, my son experimented with new dessert flavors: fennel and coriander seed in coconut milk. He asked me to taste his amazing creation. My husband was on the couch browsing YouTube videos, and I was reading my favorite Louise Penny book with a warm cup of chai tea while the dogs curled up in perpetual rest. I had a smile on my face, and I felt grateful and at peace.

Nothing life-shatteringly exciting was going on here; I was feeling the beautiful feeling of "home." Next, we made dinner together as a family. We had roast duck with butternut squash risotto and sauteed wild mushrooms—now a typical autumnal dinner at our house. I had a glass of cranberry juice with honey and spices, and I always have water with my meals. After dinner, we watched a show on Netflix together as a family and said goodnight. When I woke up in the morning, I felt refreshed and excited to face the day ahead.

I wasn't happy before and believed it was always someone else's fault. My husband was doing things that upset me, or it could be the lady at Starbucks, anyone. I didn't take responsibility for my happiness. What I learned and want to pass on to you is that no one can make us miserable. We are solely responsible for our own happiness.

I have dedicated my life to becoming the best version of myself and helping others, and I love every minute of it!

I learned through my studies that nutrition is not just for the body. It is equally essential for us to include healthy choices for the mind and soul to achieve a balanced, healthy state.

What started this whole journey was self-love. I didn't like where I was in my life, and I decided that I was worthy of finding something different and better, that I was worthy of happiness.

Now in my fifties, I live the life of my dreams. I am more excited about life than ever before. I am healthy. I learned to manage my digestive issues and learned what makes me feel best. I've started doing art again, I look and feel better than ever, and I am thrilled to pass on what I have learned to you.

Since becoming a health practitioner, I have been able to help people find their way to a happy, healthy, and fulfilling life through nutrition, art, and hypnotherapy. I have discovered through my journey that helping others makes me happiest and is food for my soul.

This book has three sections: Mind, Body, and Soul. Each focuses on practices that create balance in these areas. You will learn from reading this book that *you* can have a life that you love, a life that makes you jump out of bed in the morning because you're excited to live it. Together, we will begin a journey leading you to feel fabulous and love your life more than ever, regardless of age.

When you read the chapters of this book, I want it to be a journey for *you*. Therefore, there is no need to read them in order. Instead, look at the chapters and recipes list, and notice what jumps out. Then, make your way through in your own order, listening to what speaks to you, guided by your intuition.

If you take one thing from this book, I hope it will be to live your life through a journey of self-love and self-compassion. Amazing things happen when we discover how to find and nourish our strengths and gifts. In this book, you will find helpful tools for creating and nurturing a life of self-love, health, meaning, and purpose. I invite you to open up to the possibility of having a healthier, more intentional life. I hope you accept the invitation.

Acknowledgements

I would like to thank my husband, Aki, and son Mak, my sisters, Kelly and Tammy, and my many amazing women friends—there are too many to list here, but you know who you are—for supporting me and helping me through this journey. Their dedication means so much to me.

I would also like to thank my longtime friend, Phil Whitmarsh, at Redbrush for believing in this project and walking through every step with me. His insightful feedback and constant encouragement have transformed my words into the book you now hold in your hands. His contribution has been invaluable, and I am deeply grateful.

Contents

INTRODUCTION
Mind ~ Body ~ Soul Connection 1

MIND
Right Thinking 3
Mindfulness: The Power of Now 7
   Mindful Breathing 7
   Thirty-Second Mindfulness Meditation ... 8
   Mindful Eating 8
   Mindful Walking 9

BODY
Personalized Nutrition—
What Does Your Body Tell You? 10
Real Food 13
   The 2024 Dirty Dozen 15
   The Clean Fifteen 15
Alcohol 16
Fabulous Fats 18
Sweet Sugar 21
The Importance of Movement 25
   Walking 26
   Yoga Stretching 27
Sensational Sleep 28
   Get Natural Light during the Day 29
   Keep a Consistent Sleep Schedule 30
   Watch Caffeine Intake 30
   Time Meals 30
   Eat Healthily 30
   Avoid Alcohol before Bedtime 31
   Maximize Sleeping Environment 31

SOUL
Self-Love 33
   Self-Compassion 35
   Releasing Self-Doubt 35
   Building Self-Worth 36
Relationships 40

Trust 41
Communication in Relationships 42
Common Communication Challenges
in Relationships 42
   Intimacy 43
Spirituality 45

THE RECIPES
Bowls 49
Dragon Fruit (Pitaya) Smoothie Bowl 50
Spring Roll Bowl 52
Spicy Hawaiian Salmon Bowl 54
Salads, Soup, and More 57
Tropical Fruit Salad 58
(No added sugar) 58
Shrimp and Mango Salad 60
Blood Orange, Fennel,
and Burrata Salad 62
Microgreens salad 64
Lemon and Chickpea Soup 66
Butternut Squash Soup with Wild
Mushrooms and Miso 68
Pear and Goat Cheese appetizer 70
Tomato Tart 72
Wild Mushrooms and Creamy Polenta ... 74
Spring Herb Frittata 76
Mocktails 79
Rose Lemon Sparkler 80
Strawberry Lemonade 82
Earl Grey Citrus Mocktail 84
Yogurt 87
Yogurt Banana Split 88
Blistered Cherry Tomatoes and Yogurt 90
Strawberry Yogurt Popsicles 92
Toppings & Add-ins 95
Coconut Macadamia Nut Granola 97
Autumn Spiced Pear and Fig Compote, with
Raisins and Pecans 99

Christine Crawford

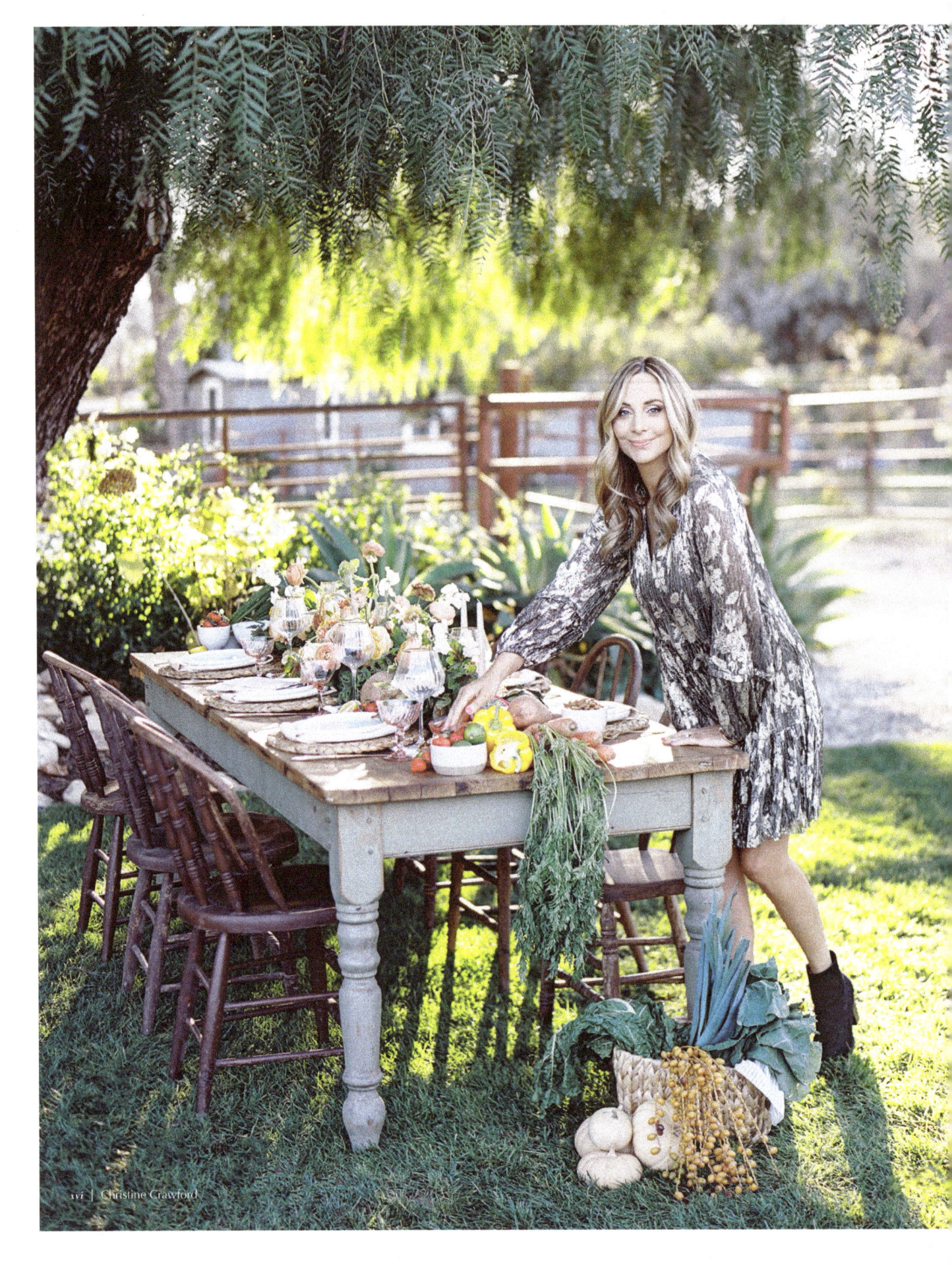

INTRO

Mind / Body / Soul Connection

> *Health is a state of complete physical, mental and social well-being, and not merely the absence of disease or infirmity. The enjoyment of the highest attainable standard of health is one of the fundamental rights of every human being.*
> —***World Health Organization 1948***

When we think about health, the first things that come to mind are a healthy diet and lots of exercise. However, our physical bodies are not the only factors affecting our health and well-being. Our minds and bodies, as well as our souls, are interconnected, and each plays a significant role in our overall health.

Most systems of medicine throughout the world treated the mind, body, and soul as a unified entity until three hundred years ago. In the seventeenth century, however, the Western world changed this view. The body and mind were seen as separate entities with no connection whatsoever to each other or the spiritual world.

Although this Western viewpoint was helpful in advancing research into pharmaceuticals and surgery, it served to decrease research into the mind-body-soul connection and their inherent ability to work together to heal.

In the last century, this has started to change. Many health professionals and researchers are now studying the mind-body connection and finding evidence of interaction among psychological, social, and biological factors in determining our state of well-being. But how do these factors achieve their impact on us? Let's break it down.

The mind is made up of mental states, such as thoughts, emotions, beliefs, attitudes, and images. Because the nervous, endocrine, and immune systems share a common chemical language, this allows different mental states to affect our biological functioning through hormones and neurotransmitters.[1]

What we think and the emotions caused by these thoughts have a significant impact on our physical and mental well-being. Negativity makes us sick. If negative thoughts and feelings are repressed, they can become feelings of hopelessness and despair.

Developing chronic stress through feelings of helplessness throws off our hormonal balance and interferes with our immune system. It also depletes the brain chemicals required for happiness.

Hormonal imbalances lead to health conditions such as hypertension, cardiovascular disease, digestive disorders, and infection.

These are just a few ways our minds and bodies affect each other.

You may wonder if you are physically, emotionally, socially, and spiritually healthy. If you are not sure, here are some questions to ask yourself.

- How is your diet? What kinds of foods do you eat?
- Are you physically healthy, or do you suffer from pain or a chronic condition?
- Are you emotionally balanced, or do you sometimes suffer from anxiety or depression?
- How much sleep do you get? Is it enough?
- How do you feel about your work? Does it give you a sense of purpose, or is it a tiring chore?
- Do you smoke, drink, or take drugs, prescription or otherwise?
- How is your energy level? Do you feel fresh and alert, or are you often fatigued?

Being mindful and taking an active role in our lives regularly is an act of profound kindness and love toward ourselves and the world. In this act of kindness, we stop scurrying around in trance-inducing busyness, which causes us to move through these moments without actually living in them.

If we can learn to see through the noise in our minds and around us, even momentarily, we will be able to live our lives fully and with integrity.

We are made of energy.

When our energy is low, we become sick. Many things affect our energy, but the most important things are

- the thoughts we think;
- the food we eat;
- the company we keep;
- the air we breathe; and
- the water we drink.

---

1 Kafaji, Talib. 2020. *The Psychology Behind Wellness and Illness: Why Do People Get Sick?* Singapore: Partridge Pub.

MIND

Right Thinking (Train Your Brain)

> *To enjoy good health, to bring true happiness to one's family, to bring peace to all, one must first discipline and control one's own mind.*
> —*Gautama Buddha*

"The sky is not the limit; your belief system is." It's hard to say who said this popular quote first, but it justly describes our human condition. If we draw the wrong conclusions about who we are, we limit what we can do and be.

Our minds are powerful. However, most of us spend little time examining the way we think. We let our thoughts control us instead of looking at what we think about and taking control of it. Thinking about our thoughts is a crucial habit to cultivate because the way we think about ourselves and the world around us turns into our reality. We can train our minds to think better. The act of thinking differently on a regular basis changes our brains physically through neuroplasticity, the ability of the brain to form and reorganize synaptic connections.

We tend to live based on stories we tell ourselves and continually reinforce. We create internal movies by focusing on specific images and thoughts while filtering out others. These images and thoughts form together to become what we perceive as our realities. We spend much time collecting information and images to support our stories.

Most of us unconsciously think the same thoughts and visualize the same mental images. Some of those can be negative. For example:

"This is never going to end."

"I never get what I want."

"I'm so unlucky."

When we do this, we continue to watch the same movie in our minds, creating and living the same quality of life.

We make decisions based on our thoughts. Our thoughts decide how we move in this world, and our actions proceed from our thoughts. By becoming aware of this, we can change our life's events and circumstances by changing our habitual thoughts.

We are not taught to control our thoughts at school and usually not at home either. Scientists are just learning of the importance of thoughts in our daily lives. The battle for control over our thoughts is real, and we can win it. We are not our thoughts. We are much bigger than they are. We need to be the director, not the follower, of our thoughts. We have the power to change the thoughts and images in our minds. It is the equivalent of inserting a new memory stick into our brain's drive.

"That sounds great, but how can I be the director of my thoughts?" you might ask.

The first thing that we need to consider is which thoughts are helpful for us and which are not.

If you are like most people, you spend much time thinking and worrying about the future and ruminating over past events. As these types of thoughts help manage our lives, they can also cause many problems. While we are entertaining negative thoughts, we cannot enjoy experiences in the now, which causes us to feel drained, anxious, and depressed.

Negativity disrupts our ability to perceive, remember, and create new neural connections, while happiness enhances our ability to be more productive and cognitively alert.

According to Teresa Aubele, PhD, and Susan Reynolds in a *Psychology Today* article titled "Happy Brain, Happy Life," "Happy people are more creative, solve problems faster, and tend to be more mentally alert."[2]

Jane E. Brody, a health columnist for *The New York Times*, writes, "Studies have shown an indisputable link between having a positive outlook and health benefits like lower blood pressure, less heart disease, better weight control, and healthier blood sugar levels."[3]

Here's how we can control negative thoughts. I have practiced these steps, and over time I have learned to keep my mind positive, even in some of the worst situations.

---

2 Reynolds, Susan, and Teresa Aubele. 2011. "Happy Brain, Happy Life." *Psychology Today* (August 2). Retrieved from https://www.psychologytoday.com/us/blog/prime-your-gray-cells/201108/happy-brain-happy-life.

3 Brody, J. E. 2017. "A Positive Outlook May Be Good for Your Health." *The New York Times* (March 27). Retrieved February 12, 2023, from https://www.nytimes.com/2017/03/27/well/live/positive-thinking-may-improve-health-and-extend-life.html.

- Develop the awareness that a thought is just a thought.
    a. Most of us have grown up to believe that we are our thoughts. We accept our thoughts unconditionally, without looking at them before we accept them as true. For example, I think, "I'm a boring person and a total failure." And what follows is the feeling and additional thought, "That's depressing." As we can't see our minds, we tend to default to this simplistic logic. We need to step outside ourselves and look at our thoughts from the perspective of an objective observer.
    b. Our thoughts are events that can be directly observed. They are influenced by many factors, such as what we ate for breakfast, what we watched on Netflix last night, different physical states such as health and hormones, and many more. They are learned from childhood and become habits through association and repetition. They are automatic subconscious behaviors. Just as a new swimmer can't become an Olympic athlete overnight, we can't stop these thought cycles without practice and effort.
    c. How we react to our thoughts is key. When we focus on our thoughts, we can see that they are all over the place, and we might feel lost. When we focus on our breathing and how our body feels, we will notice that our thoughts come and go, like passing clouds in the sky. We can look at them and see that they are just thoughts and that we do not need to have an attachment to any of them. We can then choose which thoughts we want to connect with.

- Notice your negative thoughts. If you have a hard time noticing them, consider journaling.
    a. Look for thoughts that make you feel discouraged or sad, like seeing little mistakes as failings or believing small problems are bigger than they are. Consider using a thought diary to help break down your thought process. A great thought diary app is CBT Thought Diary, available on Apple App Store and Google Play.
    b. When you identify the unhealthy thought, replace it by repeating something positive to yourself. For example, if you catch yourself saying, "This day is terrible," say, "The day may have started off hard, but it's getting better." Never say something to yourself that you wouldn't say to a friend. Keep reminding yourself to stay positive. It will eventually become a habit if you repeatedly catch yourself and replace your thoughts.

- Notice your vocabulary.
    a. Many of us speak to ourselves in absolute terms. For example, "I will *never* be able to do this," "I have the *worst* luck." When we use these absolute terms, we

exclude the chance for interpretation or explanation. Instead, say something like, "It will take some time to do this, but it will be worth the effort," or "I might have received the short end of the stick, but it's just a numbers game, and my luck will turn around."

    b. When it comes to your vocabulary, pay attention to what you say to others, as well as what you say to yourself.

- Use statements of gratitude. When you catch yourself in a negative thought, add a statement of gratitude. Instead of "I have the *worst* luck," say, "I am so grateful that I was chosen to compete as a finalist; my luck will turn around." Imagine your laptop went on the fritz, forcing you to drop it off with a tech squad. Switch up your perspective: "While this may be a small inconvenience, it allowed me to grab a cup of tea and enjoy the warm sunshine and flowers in my garden."

Mindfulness: The Power of Now

Mindfulness focuses on the present moment while calmly recognizing and accepting our feelings, thoughts, and sensations.

The human mind needs nourishing thoughts, just as the body needs proper nourishment. And like the body, the mind requires rest.

Being mindful means living in the present moment and focusing on what is happening right now, not thinking about the past or future. When focusing on the present moment, we are in touch with reality. We are aware of what is happening around us in our minds, bodies, and emotions. Anxiety resides in the future, depression resides in the past, and calmness and peace of mind live in the present.

When we are mindful, we become observers of what is happening without judgment or thinking; we are just observing. Through mindfulness, we expand our awareness, taking us to a place beyond just getting by, where we see differently, flourish, and live a more fulfilling life.

To develop mindfulness, we must be objective observers without preconceived ideas and emotions clouding our vision.

Look at these mindfulness practices to help you live more in the moment. Choose the ones that engage your attention.

Mindful Breathing

This practice couldn't be easier and brings calmness and focus. You can do this anywhere you are. You simply take ten to thirty seconds to observe your breathing. Stop what you're doing and take a few breaths, focusing on inhaling and exhaling. You can do it standing but sitting or lying down is ideal. Then resume what you were doing. That's it.

When we take mindful breaths, we interrupt the continuation of our thoughts. You will be surprised at the refreshing feeling each time you do it. This technique is also an excellent tool for dealing with stress and anxiety.

Thirty-Second Mindfulness Meditation

I enjoy meditation but don't always have time to do it for ten minutes or more when I need immediate relief. I practice the thirty-second mindful meditation daily if I remember; when I don't, I feel less at ease.

Sit up with your back straight and feet on the ground. Close your eyes and focus on your breathing. Notice the sounds and smells around you. Notice the temperature of the air. If a thought comes to your mind, acknowledge it, and imagine it floating away through the top of your head. Continue this for thirty seconds to a minute, and notice the serenity and calm it brings you.

Mindful Eating

Mindful eating is being attentive to our food in many ways, such as buying, preparing, serving, and consuming it. It is about creating a new relationship with food. Mindful eating encourages us to listen to the wisdom of our bodies instead of the often less-than-kind voices in our heads. It allows us to be calm before and during a meal to be fully present for the experience. In mindful eating, we pay attention to the present moment and use all our senses to savor the food's smells, tastes, and textures. When there is no awareness of our bodies, we can't follow their cues for hunger and fullness, causing us to eat beyond the point of satiety. When mindful of our eating, we slow down and focus on the moment as we eat. We begin to savor our food like a connoisseur. We can then enjoy our meal, experiencing the sustenance that comes from paying attention to our actions.

- Mindful eating begins with your shopping list. When making your list, think about each item you want to add to your list. Ask yourself, "Is this item good for me? Will it make me feel good after I eat it?" Try to get the bulk of your items from the produce area, avoiding the processed foods in the center aisles.

- When cooking, pay attention to the smells and sounds of the cooking process, like the sound of the knife chopping, the rinsing of the vegetables, and the sizzling of the food in the pan. Notice the aroma of the food as it changes throughout the cooking process.
- It's important to eat when hungry. Try to stagger your eating so that when you come to the table, you are hungry but not starving. If you are too hungry, you may eat ravenously, simply trying to fill the void rather than savoring your food.
- Take a small portion to start with. You can always get more later. We tend to finish what is on our plate, even when we are full before it's gone.
- When taking a bite, make sure it's small enough to move around in your mouth and take in the textures, aromas, and tastes. Notice how it feels in your mouth.
- Try to eat slowly and chew your food thoroughly to notice all the nuances in flavor and texture.

Mindful Walking

Mindful walking is another of my favorite mindfulness practices. It is a fantastic way to achieve mental clarity and calm. You can walk anywhere—in a busy city, a shopping mall, or an airport. If you can get out and walk in nature, it's even better. Studies have shown that spending time in nature can boost attention levels and has the most significant decrease in cortisol levels compared to city walking. All it takes is as little as five to ten minutes a day.

In the same way mindful breathing focuses on the breath, mindful walking focuses on the walk, paying attention to every step and noticing the movement of limbs and torso.

During mindful walking, we focus less on the destination and more on the journey. We want to avoid "zoning out" and instead notice what is happening in the moment.

As you slow down your pace, notice how the mind follows. If your mind should wander, bring your focus back to your walking. Notice the trees and how they smell. Notice how the sunshine or breeze feels on your face and body. Notice the creatures in the trees and flying in the air. When you notice these things, feel appreciation for them. When we appreciate these things, a routine walk to the market becomes a restorative mindfulness session for the mind, body, and soul.

BODY

To enjoy a healthy body, there are only a few essential elements we must employ: healthy food, healthy exercise, healthy breathing, and a healthy environment. In this section of the book, we will explore simple ways to incorporate these elements into our everyday lives.

Personalized Nutrition: What Does Your Body Tell You?

If you are like the millions of Americans trying to create a healthy life, you have likely tried at least one of the fad diets that incessantly pop up.

Personalized nutrition suggests there is no one-size-fits-all diet. Each person is unique, with distinct dietary needs and requirements. Differences in age, body composition, gender, ethnicity, size, lifestyle, and metabolism influence our overall health and the foods that make us feel best. That's why no single diet or way of eating works for everyone. The specific foods and ways of eating that make me feel good and create balance in my body may cause another person to gain weight and feel sick or lethargic.

In 2019, the results of a large-scale nutrition study showed that

> [i] Individual responses to the same foods are unique, even between identical twins, demonstrating that one-size-fits-all dietary guidelines are too simplistic. This large-scale nutrition research project was born out of the Twins UK Study—a 25-year investigation of health and lifestyle in 14,000 twins led by Tim Spector, Scientific Founder of ZOE, Professor of Genetic Epidemiology at King's College London, and author of The Diet Myth.[4]

---

4 Brody, J. E. 2017. "A Positive Outlook May Be Good for Your Health." *The New York Times* (March 27). Retrieved February 12, 2023, from https://www.nytimes.com/2017/03/27/well/live/positive-thinking-may-improve-health-and-extend-life.html.

The results of this study suggest that individual variances in the gut microbiome, exercise, metabolism, and mealtime are as significant as the composition of foods. This supports the idea that simple nutritional labeling is inadequate for assessing food.

Instead of providing broad guidelines such as "eat at least six portions of fruits and vegetables daily" or "eat two portions of oily fish per week," a personalized nutrition approach uses individual-specific information to formulate specialized advice and support relevant to the individual.

Having worked one-on-one with clients, I have come to realize that personalized nutrition is the key to achieving our healthiest state of being. I have observed and experienced that no one way of eating is the best for everyone. Yet medicine and science are constantly searching for the magic pill—the perfect way of eating to solve all humanity's diet-related problems. Fortunately, the scientific world is now beginning to see that a personalized approach to diet is beneficial.

It's time to recognize our individuality. There is no one way of eating that will always work for us. Foods we've eaten for years may no longer agree with us and cause us distress as we age. It's important to eat intuitively, trusting our bodies to guide us to the foods that best support our needs rather than getting stuck in dietary dogma.

There are now many tests you can take that will tell you about your genetic makeup and what foods will be most beneficial to you. The bad news is that they are expensive because the technology is new. Fortunately, we already have free twenty-four-hour access to the world's most sophisticated laboratory: we're living in it. Our bodies are highly intelligent biocomputers that have evolved helpful instincts to keep us alive and well.

Bloating, exhaustion, and weight gain are all signs that something we are eating or how we are eating isn't working for us. Listening to our bodies' messages before they become unbearable can prevent many chronic illnesses, doctor visits, medications, and operations. Using an elimination diet to remove foods that we believe are causing our bodies distress is a great way to narrow down the suspects.

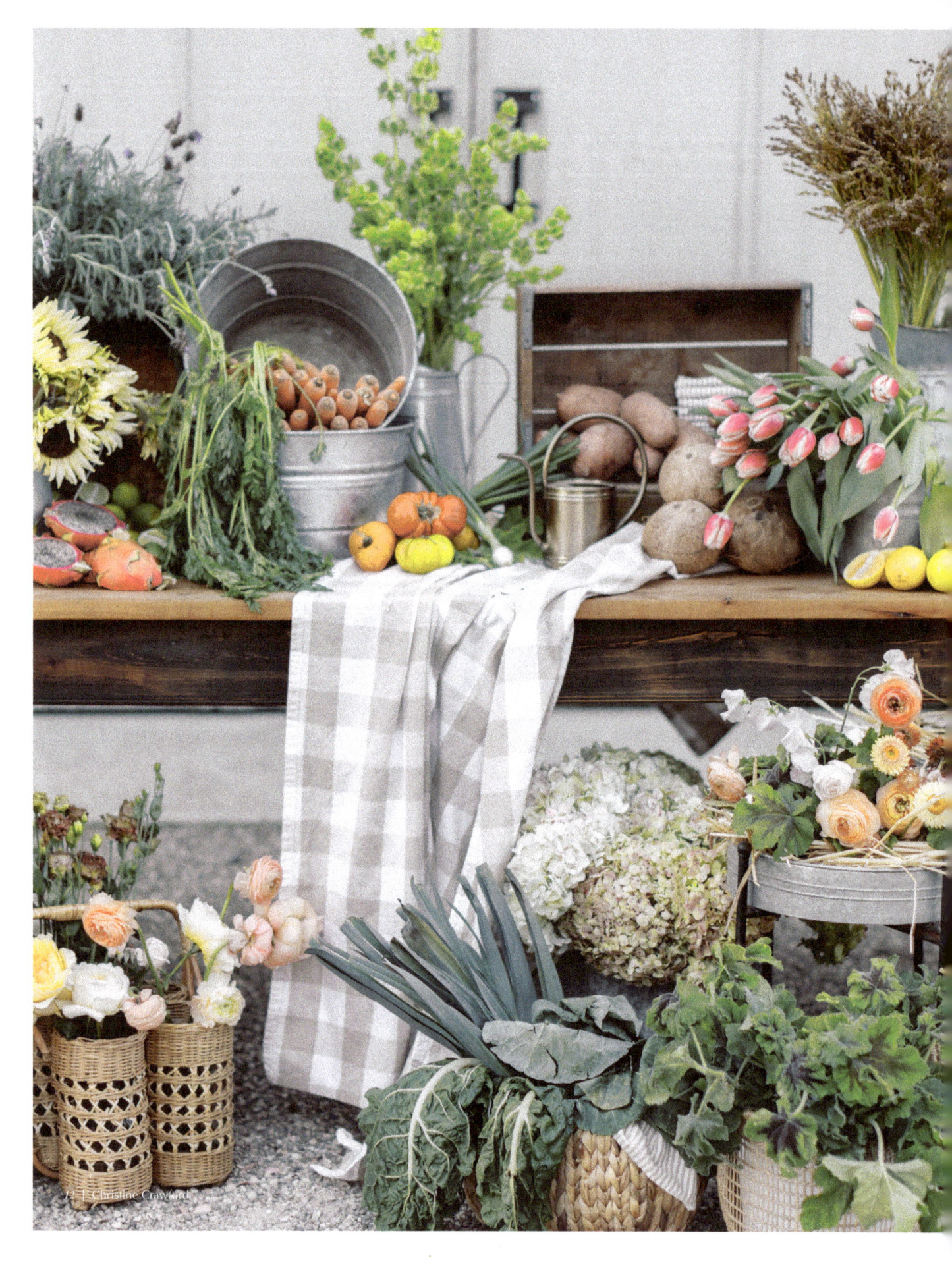

Real Food

*The food you eat can be either the safest and most powerful
form of medicine, or the slowest form of poison.*
—Ann Wigmore

A few rules surround what foods to eat that benefit most beings.

- Eat real food
- Avoid chemicals
- Avoid processed foods

What is real food?

A thing is real if it is genuine and true, not imitation or artificial. Food is a nutritious substance that supplies and nourishes us with what we need to maintain life and growth.

Real food is food in its natural and original state without alteration.

But before I bore you with what you should and shouldn't eat and loads of information and statistics, let me say that eating is a common sense sort of thing. Our bodies already know what is good for us.

Listening to our bodies is one of the most important things we can do for our physical health.

How do you feel after eating a large basket of greasy French fries? I would wager you have a tummy ache. How do you feel when you eat a *handful* of greasy French fries? Not so bad, I suppose. These are our body's cues that tell us what it needs and doesn't need.

Here are some guidelines for eating healthy, real food. Limit your foods to those with less than five ingredients, and without ingredients, you do not recognize or can't pronounce.

- Stick to the perimeter of the supermarket. The middle of the market is filled with foods with a longer shelf life than those on the perimeter, thus, are full of chemicals and preservatives.
- Don't buy food to eat in the car. Most fast-food restaurant foods are full of chemicals and nonfood ingredients.
- Eating with family and loved ones around a table is essential for savoring our food and not devouring it as fast as possible. When we eat slowly, with pleasure, and with loved ones, it benefits our digestion and our souls.

Eating whole foods the way they came into this world—to me, that is *real* food. I am not big on diet foods, especially the low-fat and fat-free foods you see on every supermarket's shelves. Low-fat foods are marketed as "healthy," but processed foods, such as low-fat yogurt, often replace the fat with unhealthy ingredients, namely sugar. Added sugar consumption is a leading contributor to many diseases of the body. We don't need to be sugar-phobic, but choosing healthier alternatives will deter cravings for more sugar and spikes in our blood glucose.

Here are ten low-fat foods that are unhealthy and packed with sugar:

1. Granola (and other low-fat breakfast cereals and bars)
2. Low-fat salad dressing
3. Protein bars
4. Turkey bacon (and other processed meats)
5. Low-fat and frozen yogurts
6. Flavored oatmeal
7. Baked potato chips
8. Bottled smoothies
9. Low-fat cereals and breads
10. Reduced-fat peanut butter

Some better choices are:

1. Homemade granola using unprocessed foods such as oats and nuts
2. Salad dressing made with olive oil, lemon, and herbs
3. Homemade protein bars using dates as a sweetener
4. Rotisserie chicken
5. Plain yogurt with unsweetened berry compote mixed in
6. Oatmeal with banana, nuts, and berries
7. Hard-boiled egg salad using plain Greek yogurt or avocado

8. Homemade smoothies with bananas as a sweetener.
9. Hummus with fresh or roasted veggies, soft-boiled egg, and cheese
10. Unsweetened, full-fat nut butter.

See The Recipes section to make these and more.

When it comes to eating, I prefer organic choices. Eating organic isn't always possible, but some foods are worth searching down the organic varieties. Below is a list of the Environmental Working Group's (EWG) Dirty Dozen and Clean Fifteen. In a press conference, the EWG said, "This year, the USDA's tests found residues of potentially harmful chemical pesticides on nearly 70 percent of the non-organic fresh produce sold in the U.S. Before testing fruits and vegetables, the USDA washes, scrubs, and peels them, as consumers would."[5] I like to follow their guidelines for which foods to eat organic.

The 2024 Dirty Dozen

These foods are the most important to eat organically:

- Strawberries
- Kale/Collard/Mustard greens
- Peaches
- Nectarines
- Bell and Hot Peppers
- Blueberries
- Spinach
- Grapes
- Pears
- Apples
- Cherries
- Green Beans

The Clean Fifteen

- Sweet Corn
- Onions
- Asparagus
- Cabbage
- Mangoes
- Avocados
- Papayas
- Honeydew Melon
- Watermelon
- Sweet Potatoes
- Pineapples
- Sweet Peas
- Kiwi
- Mushrooms
- Carrots[6]

This is not an exhaustive list but a great place to start.

---

5 Johnson, Greg. 2024. "Dirty Dozen, Clean 15 Lists Released for 2024." Blue Book Services (March 17). https://www.producebluebook.com/2021/03/17/dirty-dozen-clean-15-lists-released-for-2021/#.

6 Environmental Working Group. (n.d.). Check out @EWG's 2024 Shopper's Guide to Pesticides in Produce™! #DirtyDozen #CleanFifteen | @ewg |. https://www.ewg.org/foodnews/summary.php

Alcohol

Alcohol is ever-present in our society. We can find it almost anywhere we go. Imbibing occasionally can be enjoyable and harmless, but we need to remember that alcohol is a toxin. Alcohol is a psychoactive and dependence-producing substance and has been classified as a Group 1 carcinogen by the International Agency for Research on Cancer—this is the highest risk group, including asbestos, radiation, and tobacco. Alcohol causes at least seven types of cancer, including breast, colorectal, larynx, liver, esophagus, oral cavity, and pharynx cancers, and it is a probable cause of pancreatic cancer. Even small amounts can cause hormone imbalance, impede brain function, and stress the liver.[7]

Whether good or bad, most of us have associations with alcohol. For example, I have a social association. When I think about having a drink, I imagine being at a social function like a party and enjoying myself with friends. If you are like me and have always socialized with a drink in your hand, attending a social function without drinking can be unnerving. I also associated alcohol with reward—champagne to celebrate an anniversary, for birthdays, Christmas, you name it. If it's celebratory, the champagne should flow. At age forty, I discovered how challenging child rearing could be. So when I had my boy, I started celebrating with a glass of wine on extra tough days at 5:00 or 4:30-ish ("It's five o'clock somewhere, right?") for making it through the day. I would drink a glass of wine with dinner, and many days I would keep drinking until I crawled into bed. Not surprisingly, this started a downward spiral. Eventually, it got to the point where I'd go to sleep woozy, wake up at 3:00 a.m. from the sugar shooting back from my liver, take an hour or so to fall back asleep, and wake up again at 7:00 a.m.—or whenever my son woke me up—with a headache and general feeling of malaise. This pattern, on a daily repeat, did me in. I had to change. I've quit drinking alcohol for eight years, which was one of the best things I've ever done to feel healthy and whole. However, I think taking periodic breaks can be beneficial too.

---

[7] World Health Organization. 2023. "No Level of Alcohol Consumption Is Safe for Our Health." World Health Organization (January 4). Retrieved February 20, 2023, from https://www.who.int/europe/news/item/04-01-2023-no-level-of-alcohol-consumption-is-safe-for-our-health#:~:text=Alcohol%20is%20a%20toxic%2C%20psychoactive,includes%20asbestos%2C%20radiation%20and%20tobacco.

If you decide to take a break from alcohol, make it fun. Try and see your time away as an adventure. Focus on what you will gain, not on the absence of the drink. Ask yourself, "What shall I do with my extra time?"

Here are some ways to use your time away from alcohol.

- Instead of spending your spare time having a glass (or more) of wine, try a new activity. Is there something you've always wanted to do and haven't made time for yet? You could try a new recipe, pick up a musical instrument, paint, go for a walk, or redecorate. The list goes on. Make it your special time.
- Stir up some sensational mocktails. Recently, restaurants have had creative and exciting nonalcoholic cocktails on their menus. I have taken it upon myself to incorporate the best parts into my mocktails. You can find recipes at the end of this book.

Choosing to quit drinking for a period isn't for everyone. We are unique; what works for you or me may not work for others.

Alcohol can also affect our mood. For some, anxiety is a significant factor in choosing to drink. Alcohol can sometimes reduce anxiety, but it is only temporary until the alcohol wears off. In the long run, alcohol can cause anxiety or depression as it is a depressant.

It's important to notice signs of alcoholism or addiction. You can take a self-assessment at www.aa.org/self-assessment. In battling drug and alcohol addiction, getting help over the phone is an often-overlooked resource. The National Rehab Hotline at 866-210-1303 is free to answer your questions about alcohol addiction or help you find a local Alcoholics Anonymous group. The calls are answered by a behavioral health specialist knowledgeable about alcoholism, mental health, and recovery.

Fabulous Fats

Fat is essential in our diets, but some fats are healthier. For example, unsaturated fat is the most beneficial type of fat. Dr. Walter Willett of Harvard School of Public Health says, "Eating unsaturated fat in place of refined grains and sugar can improve blood cholesterol profiles and lower triglycerides, and in turn, lower the risk of heart disease."[8]

Unsaturated fat raises our HDL or "good cholesterol" levels. We can find it in plants and oily fish. Examples are olive oil, seeds, nuts, avocado, and salmon. Saturated fat is not as healthy, but a small amount of saturated fat is okay. We can't avoid it entirely because foods with healthy fats often have a small amount of saturated fat.

"Your body needs a regular fat intake," says Vasanti Malik, a research scientist with the Department of Nutrition at Harvard's T. H. Chan School of Public Health. "Fat helps give your body energy, protects your organs, supports cell growth, keeps cholesterol and blood pressure under control, and helps your body absorb vital nutrients. When you focus too much on cutting out all fat, you can deprive your body of what it needs most."[9]

While fat has often been vilified in the past, it is essential to recognize that not all fats are created equal. In fact, monounsaturated and polyunsaturated fats are highly beneficial for our bodies. These healthy fats provide essential nutrients and energy and contribute to various vital functions.

Fat serves as a concentrated source of energy. It provides more than twice the amount of energy per gram compared to carbohydrates or proteins. This energy reserve is significant during prolonged physical exertion or when our body needs a readily available fuel source. Fat acts as a backup fuel that can be used when carbohydrates are depleted, ensuring a steady supply of energy.

---

8 Willett, Walter, and Amy Miller. 2018. "Ask the Expert: Healthy Fats." The Nutrition Source (July 24). Retrieved February 12, 2023, from https://www.hsph.harvard.edu/nutritionsource/2012/06/21/ask-the-expert-healthy-fats/.

9 Harvard Health Publishing, Harvard Medical School. (2021). "Know the Facts about Fats." Harvard Health (April 19). Retrieved February 12, 2023, from https://www.health.harvard.edu/staying-healthy/know-the-facts-about-fats.

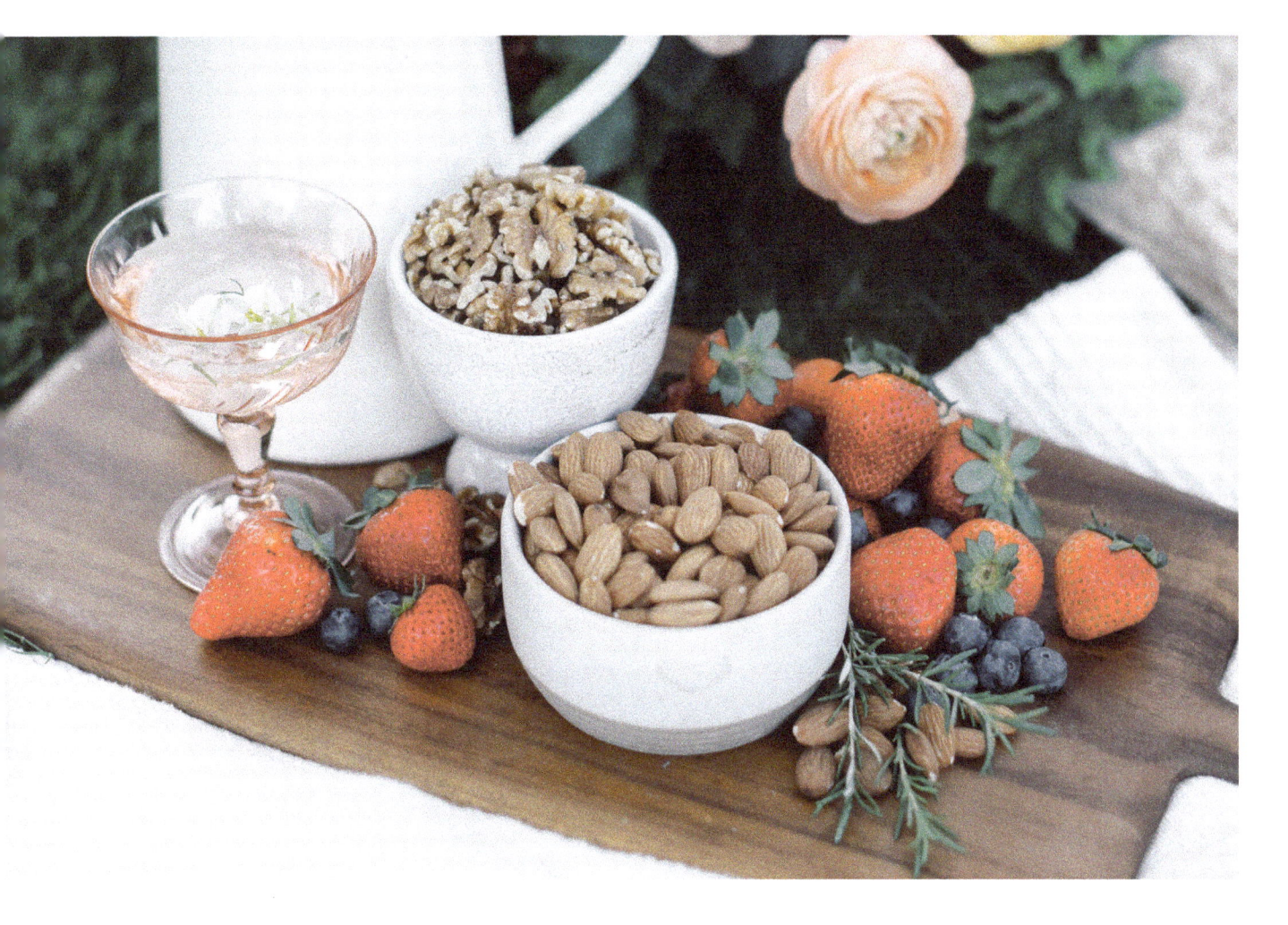

Furthermore, dietary fat aids the absorption of fat-soluble vitamins (A, D, E, and K), which are crucial for various bodily functions. These vitamins are necessary for maintaining healthy skin, promoting bone health, supporting immune function, and aiding in blood clotting. The presence of fat in our diet helps facilitate the absorption and transportation of these essential vitamins, ensuring they can be utilized effectively by our bodies.

Healthy fats are also involved in the production of hormones, including sex hormones such as estrogen and testosterone. These hormones are vital for reproductive health, regulating the menstrual cycle, and maintaining optimal sexual function. Additionally, fat helps insulate and protect vital organs, acts as a cushioning agent, and supports healthy cell membranes.

Saturated and trans fats in processed foods should be limited due to their potential adverse effects on heart health. On the other hand, unsaturated fats, like those found in avocados, nuts, seeds, and olive oil, are healthier options.

See the recipes section for dishes made with healthy fats.

Tropical Fruit Salad

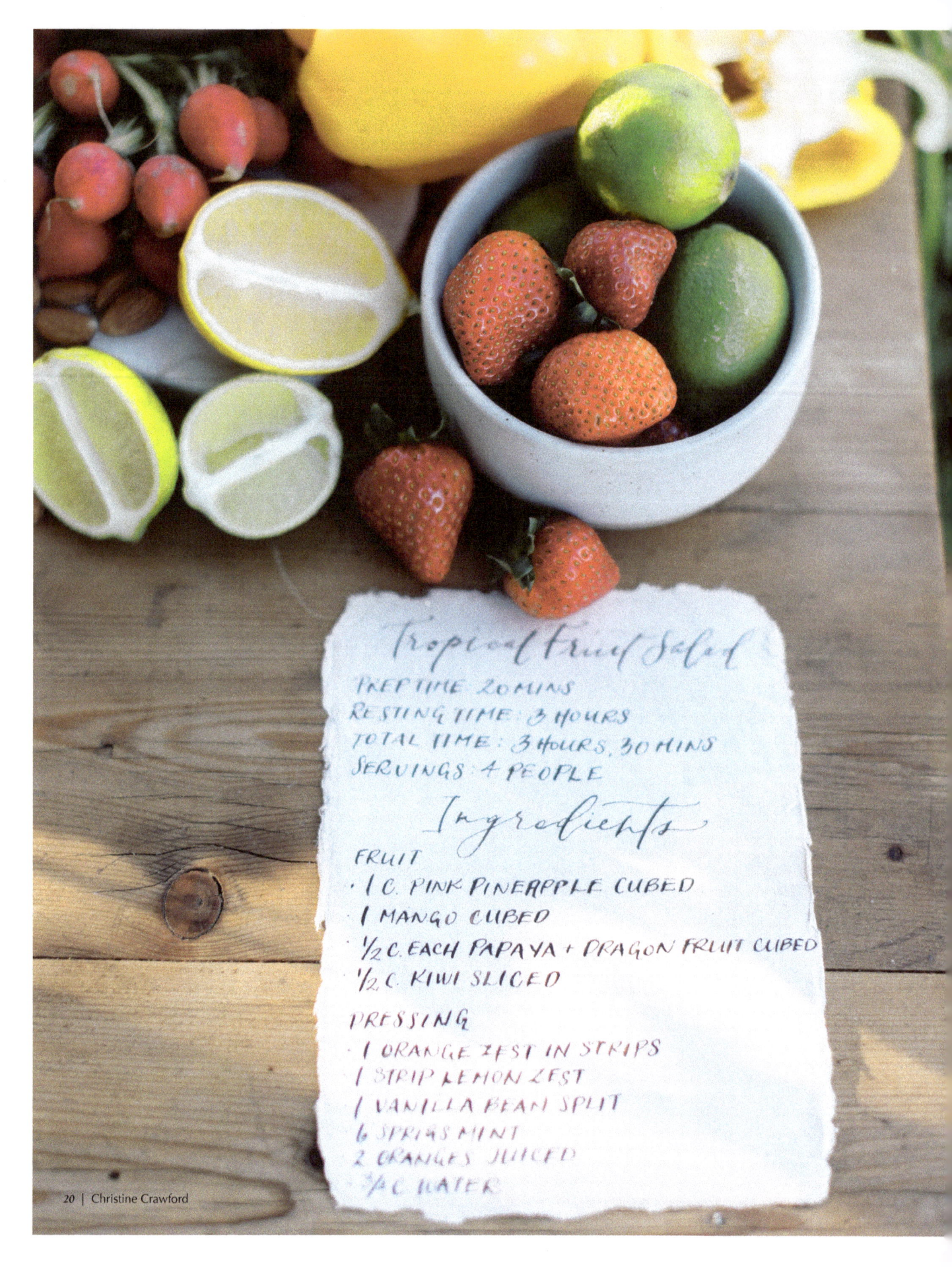

PREP TIME: 20 MINS
RESTING TIME: 3 HOURS
TOTAL TIME: 3 HOURS, 30 MINS
SERVINGS: 4 PEOPLE

Ingredients

FRUIT
- 1 C. PINK PINEAPPLE CUBED
- 1 MANGO CUBED
- ½ C. EACH PAPAYA + DRAGON FRUIT CUBED
- ½ C. KIWI SLICED

DRESSING
- 1 ORANGE ZEST IN STRIPS
- 1 STRIP LEMON ZEST
- 1 VANILLA BEAN SPLIT
- 6 SPRIGS MINT
- 2 ORANGES JUICED
- ¾ C. WATER

Sweet Sugar

Being a nutrition consultant, I am acutely aware of the numerous reasons to limit refined sugar consumption. But not all sugar is bad for us. For example, naturally occurring sugars, such as those in fruit, vegetables, and grains, supply us with the glucose that gives our bodies the energy we need to function. Unfortunately, added sugars create havoc in our bodies. Added sugar is any sugar that manufacturers or we add to our food to make it taste better or extend its shelf-life.

When considering the role of added sugar in your life, ask yourself, "How do I feel after having consumed added sugar?" "How do I feel fifteen to thirty minutes after consuming refined sugar?" If you are like me, you feel great for the first fifteen minutes, then start to feel lethargic. I proceed to feel jittery and unfocused with heart palpitations. Not long after that, I crave salty foods, and after I have satisfied the salty urge, I start to crave sugary foods again. For me, it is a roller coaster. I overeat and feel exhausted and depleted by the end of the day. When I consume sugar in fruit or other naturally occurring sugars in their whole form, I don't experience the sugar/salt rollercoaster.

Whole foods with naturally occurring sugars, such as apples and grapefruit, also contain dietary fiber. We digest these foods more slowly, and there is a healthy steady supply of sugar to the body. On the other hand, foods with refined sugars, such as candy bars and sugary drinks, have little to no fiber, allowing sugar to move quickly through the bloodstream. This quick sugar travel is why we experience a sugar high and crash after consuming sugary treats.

When I choose to eat added sugar, it is a special occasion, not the norm. However, I like to use palm sugar (sometimes called coconut sugar) or maple syrup. I use them instead of table sugar because they have a lower glycemic index than cane sugar, releasing the sugar into the system more slowly. If you want to incorporate maple syrup into your diet, check that it is 100% maple syrup to ensure it is low glycemic.

I also love to use pure fruit and berry juice as a sweetener. It has a mellow sweetness and contains vitamins and minerals unavailable in cane sugar, which has no nutrients. I have berries in the freezer at all times. I take a combination of berries and microwave them until they release their juices, about a minute. I use this berry juice on pancakes, smoothies, and any place you use syrup. If you want to bring out the sweetness more, simmer the juices until they have reduced by about half, and you will have a thicker, sweeter version. Fruit and berry compotes are a fabulous way to add natural sweetness to any dish. Bananas are also great sweeteners and have many nutritional benefits. I use them as a sweetener in smoothies, oatmeal, cakes, and bread. I have included recipes with my favorite ways to use fruit as sweeteners in the Recipes section.

It is important to consume any sweetener in moderation, especially if you have specific dietary concerns or are managing a condition such as diabetes. Pairing it with other foods with a lower GI or consuming it as part of a balanced meal can help mitigate its impact on blood sugar levels.

As always, it's advisable to consult with your doctor, who can provide personalized guidance based on your individual needs and health goals.

The Glycemic Index (GI) is a measure of how quickly carbohydrate-containing foods raise blood sugar levels. Foods with a low GI (55 or below) are digested more slowly, resulting in a slower and more gradual increase in blood sugar levels.

It is an important concept in nutrition and health for many reasons:

- It measures blood sugar. For individuals with diabetes, particularly type 2, managing blood sugar levels is crucial.
- Research suggests a diet focused on low-GI foods can improve blood lipid profiles, potentially decreasing the risk of heart disease.
- For athletes or those engaging in prolonged physical activity, understanding the GI can help choose the right foods for sustained energy. For instance, they might consume lower-GI foods for long-lasting energy, and higher-GI foods for rapid recovery post-exercise.
- There is evidence that low-GI diets can be beneficial for weight management.
- Many low-GI foods are also high in fiber, vitamins, and minerals, which are beneficial for overall health.

Here are some of the most common added sugars and their average glycemic index (GI) values:

- **Glucose (Dextrose):** 100 - Often used in food and drink processing.
- **Sucrose (Table Sugar):** 65 - This is the granulated sugar most commonly used in cooking and baking.

- **High-Fructose Corn Syrup (HFCS):** 58-65 - Commonly used in sodas, candy, and many processed foods. The GI value can vary depending on its specific formulation.
- **Honey:** 50-58 - The exact GI can vary depending on the floral source and processing.
- **Maple Syrup:** 54 - Natural sweetener from the sap of sugar maple trees.
- **Palm Sugar:** 35-50 - Derived from the sap of various species of palm tree.
- **Agave Nectar:** 10-30 - Often marketed as a natural sweetener, its GI can vary, but it is high in fructose, which gives it a lower GI. However, high fructose consumption has other health concerns.

It's essential to understand that while the glycemic index provides information on how quickly a sugar or food can raise blood glucose levels, it doesn't provide a complete picture of a food or ingredient's healthfulness. Many factors, including diet, how the sugar is consumed (e.g., with fiber or fat), and individual variations, can influence the glycemic response. Also, just because a specific type of sugar has a lower glycemic index, it doesn't mean it is "healthy," especially if consumed in large quantities.[10]

---

10 U.S. National Library of Medicine. (n.d.). Glycemic index and diabetes: *Medlineplus medical encyclopedia. MedlinePlus*. https://medlineplus.gov/ency/patientinstructions/000941.htm

24 | Christine Crawford

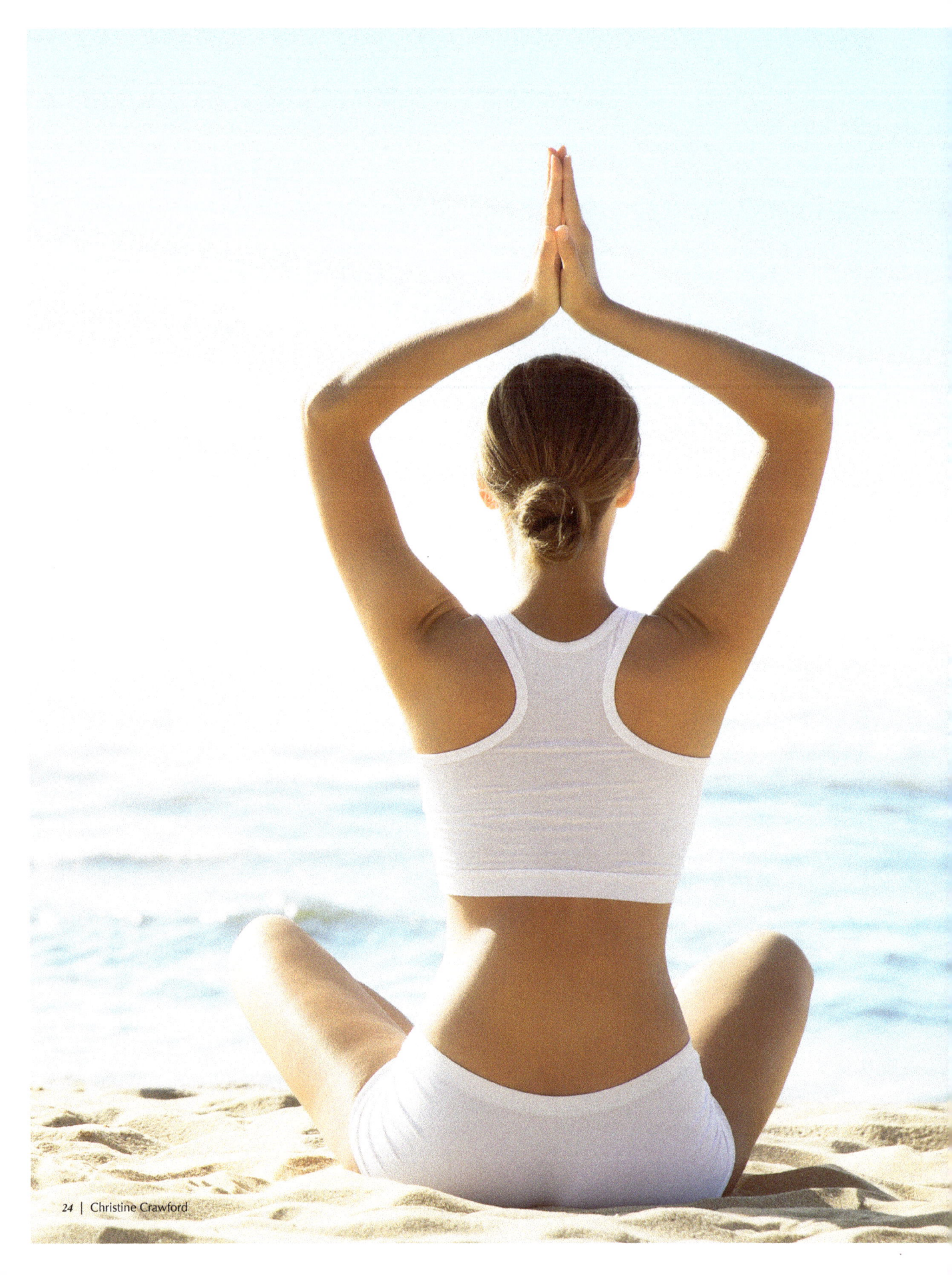

The Importance of Movement

You may remember from the beginning of the book that I suffered from digestive issues, bloating, and discomfort. I listened to my body and started cutting out foods I could not tolerate. It helped some, but unfortunately, I still struggled with bloating and discomfort, albeit less severely.

My family and I went to Amsterdam a few summers ago to support my son's jazz music endeavors. I love Europe for many reasons, but the food is one of the biggest. Since I had never been to Amsterdam, I decided to try some dishes with ingredients I was intolerant of because I wanted to experience the culture. Of course, I expected the symptoms afterward, but they never came.

When we returned to the States, I began to suffer the same symptoms as always—bloating and discomfort. I racked my brain to find some explanation for why I could splurge a little when I was in Amsterdam but not when I was in California. I listed all the differences between the two cities, and the big one that kept standing out was that we walked most places daily.

Before moving to Los Angeles, I lived in New York City, where I didn't suffer from digestive issues. In NYC, I walked everywhere for the most part. Since moving to Los Angeles, I had to accept that it was necessary to drive to most places. The city is enormous, and getting from one appointment to the other usually takes thirty to forty minutes by car. I worked out regularly, but I only walked the dog, which was sporadic, and we didn't go far.

Then, I thought about walking and how hip flexion muscles also contributed to abdominal flexion and realized that my neglect of walking might contribute to my stomach issues. So I started walking the dogs more regularly. I walked faster and farther, and guess what? My symptoms began to subside! Finally, after listening to my body, I heard. Whenever I feel digestive discomfort, I realize I haven't walked as much as I need.

After my discovery, I researched how movement affects gut health. I was surprised to learn of a recent scientific discovery that explains how gentle movement "modifies the gut microbiota, with positive health effects."[11] Microflora in our gut provides nutrients, regulates epithelial development, and improves our immune system. "The gut microbiota plays various important functions for the host's health. For example, the gut microbiota is essential for the motility of the gastrointestinal tract, facilitating peristalsis."[12] In other words, it helps the intestines facilitate wave-like muscle contractions that move food through the digestive tract. Recent findings suggest low-intensity exercise can influence the GIT, reducing the contact time between pathogens and the gastrointestinal mucus layer. As a result, experts believe gentle movement has protective effects, reducing the risk of colon cancer, diverticulosis, and inflammatory bowel disease.[13]

Moving our bodies every day is essential. It gets our blood flowing and our hearts beating and has many benefits:

- Reduced risk of heart disease
- Increased muscle strength
- Reduced body fat
- Stronger bones
- Increased heart and lung fitness
- Increased digestive function

Walking

Walking briskly for thirty minutes daily ensures health benefits; if difficult, try walking for ten minutes three times daily. Some ways to walk more are walking the dogs (my favorite), walking instead of driving, parking your car at a central location, and walking to all the shops. Also, you can start taking stairs instead of elevators or escalators or park far away from your destination and walk the rest of the way. These are just some ideas. There are endless ways to incorporate more walking into your daily schedule.

---

11 Monda, V., Villano, I., Messina, A., Valenzano, A., Esposito, T., Moscatelli, F., Viggiano, A., et al. 2017. "Exercise Modifies the Gut Microbiota with Positive Health Effects." *Oxidative Medicine and Cellular Longevity*. Retrieved February 12, 2023, from https://www.ncbi.nlm.nih.gov/pmc/articles/PMC5357536/.

12 Berg, R. D. 1996. "The Indigenous Gastrointestinal Microflora." *Trends in Microbiology* 4 (11): 430–35. doi: 10.1016/0966-842x(96)10057-3.

13 Monda, V., Villano, I., Messina, A., Valenzano, A., Esposito, T., Moscatelli, F., Viggiano, A., et al. "Exercise Modifies the Gut Microbiota with Positive Health Effects." *Oxidative Medicine and Cellular Longevity*. https://www.ncbi.nlm.nih.gov/pmc/articles/PMC5357536/.

Yoga Stretching

I am a big fan of yoga stretching. The gentle stretching releases toxins and stuck energy from stress in our lives. It allows us to treat our bodies with kindness and love. By listening and responding to our bodies this way, we focus on breathing and being present. Yoga stretching brings calmness and rejuvenation through alignment with our inner core. It improves balance, strength, and flexibility and can ease arthritis symptoms and back pain.

Working with a professional in a class setting or one-on-one is the best way to approach yoga, although you can teach yourself if you don't have any physical issues. Please consult with your physician to ensure that yoga is advisable for you.

According to Very Well Fit, the Best Yoga Apps of 2023 are

- Best Overall: Yoga Studio by Gaiam
- Best for All Fitness Levels: Down Dog
- Best for Community Support: Daily Yoga
- Best for Busy People: Glo
- Best for Kids: Simply Yoga
- Best Budget: Yoga Workout
- Best for Beginners: Pocket Yoga
- Best for the Office: 5-Minute Yoga[14]

I use Glo and enjoy it very much.

Some of my favorite yoga stretches are:

- Child's Pose
- Legs Up the Wall
- Cat and Cow Pose
- Seated Heart Opener
- Forward Fold
- Happy Baby

---

[14] Luff, C. 2023. *Best Yoga Apps of 2023.* Verywell Fit (February 9). Retrieved February 24, 2023, from https://www.verywellfit.com/best-yoga-apps-4176689.

Sensational Sleep

"Sleep services all aspects of our body in one way or another: molecular, energy balance, as well as intellectual function, alertness, and mood," says Dr. Merrill Mitler, a sleep expert and neuroscientist at the National Institute of Health.[15]

When I don't get enough sleep, I am positively miserable. I'm grumpy. I make bad decisions and inevitably anger someone. My thinking is foggy, and my reflexes are slow. Simply put, my mind and body can't function at an acceptable level.

Over the years and through my extensive training, I have learned that sleep is just as important as what we eat and how much exercise we get. Beyond physical health, emotional and mental health are equally important to a balanced and fulfilling life. Good sleep is integral to bringing all these elements together. Good sleep improves our brain efficiency, mood, and health. Not getting enough sleep raises the risk of many diseases and disorders, including heart disease, stroke, and dementia.

In 2012, researchers found a pseudo-lymphatic system in the brain called the glymphatic system. It is now known that this system flushes toxic metabolites and waste from our brains. One of the toxins it flushes is beta-amyloid. A buildup of beta-amyloid in the brain has been linked to Alzheimer's disease, and sleep has been shown to play a role in clearing beta-amyloid out of the brain. The glymphatic system constantly filters toxins from the brain, but this system is disengaged during wakefulness. It is predominantly active during slow-wave sleep stages.[16] Because of this daily clearance of metabolites, sufficient sleep is an absolute necessity.

Adults aged twenty-five and older need approximately seven to nine hours of sleep. Going to bed regularly every night allows our bodies to get into a sleep schedule, making it easier to fall asleep each night.

Short-term effects of sleep deprivation include:

---

15 National Institutes of Health. 2018. "The Benefits of Slumber." News in Health (April 4). Retrieved February 12, 2023, from https://newsinhealth.nih.gov/2013/04/benefits-slumber

16 Reddy, O. C., and Y. D. van der Werf. 2020. "The Sleeping Brain: Harnessing the Power of the Glymphatic System through Lifestyle Choices." National Library of Medicine: PMD Pub Med Central. https://www.ncbi.nlm.nih.gov/pmc/articles/PMC7698404/.

- memory, performance, and cognition deficiency;
- increased reactivity to stress;
- increased pain sensitivity;
- increased anxiety;
- emotional distress, and
- metabolic changes, increasing ghrelin (hunger hormones) and decreasing leptin (appetite-control hormone).[17]

Long-term effects of sleep deprivation include:

- increased risk of heart disease and high blood pressure, as well as type 2 diabetes;
- compromised immunity;
- increased risk of obesity. There is a 50 percent increased risk of obesity if we get five hours of sleep or less regularly; and
- increased risk for dementia, premature aging, and Alzheimer's disease.

Keeping good sleep habits can be more complicated than it sounds, and a good night's rest can often be elusive. We have all experienced the trouble of trying to fall asleep but are unable to because our minds are racing. We do the best we can, but sometimes that's not enough. Understanding our body's internal clock is essential to establishing a good sleep schedule. Our bodies have an internal clock that regulates our biological processes, including sleep, hormone levels, and more. This clock is called the circadian clock. The circadian clock, located in the hypothalamus, has thousands of neurons. It has an internally driven twenty-four-hour rhythm that resets daily by the sun's light/dark cycle. This internal body clock sets the timing for many circadian rhythms, which regulate sleep/wake cycles, hormonal activity, and eating and digesting.[18]

Here are some ways to increase the sleep you achieve each night.

Get Natural Light during the Day

Darkness and light trigger our circadian rhythm. Therefore, getting enough natural light during the day and less light at night is essential to keep our circadian rhythm in sync with the external environment.

---

17 IIN. 2021. "Sleep Is the Most Important Thing for Your Brain and Body: Nine Steps to Optimize Your Sleep." Institute for Integrative Nutrition (March 23). Retrieved February 12, 2023, from https://www.integrativenutrition.com/blog/nine-steps-to-optimize-your-sleepn.

18 National Institute for Occupational Safety and Health (NIOSH). 2020. "Circadian Rhythms and Circadian Clock." Centers for Disease Control and Prevention (April 1). https://www.cdc.gov/niosh/emres/longhourstraining/clock.html.

Keep a Consistent Sleep Schedule

Keeping a consistent sleep schedule helps keep the circadian rhythm in check. According to a National Institute of Health study, adherence to a structured sleep schedule results in regular sleep timing and improved alignment between sleep and circadian timing.[19] Blood pressure, heart rate, and cardiovascular operations depend on the circadian rhythm to remain healthy. Creating a regular sleep schedule improves quality sleep, leading to a lower risk of disease, better immune function, increased performance, better emotional well-being, and more.[20]

Watch Caffeine Intake

All of us metabolize caffeine differently. I must stop drinking caffeine around 6:00 p.m. to get a good night's sleep. Your situation may be different. Pay attention to the times you consume caffeine and how it affects your sleep. Coffee, tea, soda, and chocolate contain caffeine. Some medications also contain caffeine, so read the labels.

Time Meals

Nutrition, metabolism, and circadian rhythms are intricately linked. For example, insulin, a hormone created by our bodies to regulate blood sugar, has been shown to act as a "timing signal" for our cells. When we eat, we release insulin, so we must eat regularly for our body's timing to stay consistent. Also, eating too close to bedtime means our bodies are busy digesting while sleeping, which can cause sleep disturbance. Therefore, doctors recommend eating our last meal at least three hours before bed to give our bodies time to digest and send proper signals to wind down.

Eat Healthily

The same foods that promote overall health are also the best for good sleep. Avoid processed foods, including sugar, and eat a balanced diet with quality protein, fruits, vegetables, healthy fats, and whole grains.

---

19 McMahon, W. R., S. Ftouni, A. J. K. Phillips, C. Beatty, S. W. Lockley, S. M. W. Rajaratnam, P. Maruff, S. P. A. Drummond, and C. Anderson. 2020. "The Impact of Structured Sleep Schedules Prior to an In-Laboratory Study: Individual Differences in Sleep and Circadian Timing." PLoS One 15 (8): e0236566. doi: 10.1371/journal.pone.0236566.

20 National Institutes of Health. 2018. "The Benefits of Slumber." *News in Health* (April). Retrieved February 12, 2023, from https://newsinhealth.nih.gov/2013/04/benefits-slumber.

Avoid Alcohol before Bedtime

Many believe alcohol helps them sleep well because it makes them feel tired and fall asleep more quickly. But unfortunately, as the body metabolizes the alcohol, a period of arousal causes us to wake up. According to the Sleep Foundation, drinking before bed often causes disruptions later in the sleep cycle as liver enzymes metabolize alcohol. This can lead to a host of problems, including daytime sleepiness.[21]

Maximize Sleeping Environment

- **Keep your bedroom space for sleeping and sex only.** Don't watch tv or use your computer or phone in your bedroom. Doing other activities may cause an association with them. Likewise, keep stimulating conversations (e.g., marital discussions) out of the room, lest we lie awake worrying about them.

- **Keep all electronics out of your bedroom.** Just as we want to keep the stimulating conversation out of our rooms, keeping stimulating electronics out is vital. The content might keep us awake, as it is adrenalizing, but the light they emit also mimics daylight and can trick our circadian rhythm into believing it's daylight. This can cause our systems to delay the release of melatonin, one of the hormones that help us sleep. If you use your phone as an alarm, set it far from your bed. Having it too close makes it tempting to continuously check it for texts, emails, or social media notifications.

- **Keep your bedroom dark and quiet.** Light can disrupt the circadian rhythm. If you can't keep the room dark, wear a sleep mask and avoid glowing electronics. If you cannot avoid noise, try using a white noise machine or fan to help block out sounds.

- **Keep your bedroom cool.** Our body temperature needs to drop to prepare for sleep. Keeping the room between sixty and sixty-seven degrees helps the process.

- **Make your bed cozy and inviting.** If your mattress is older than nine years, it's time to replace it. Comfortable pillows, bedding, and mattresses will help you get a good night's sleep.

Tackling great sleeping habits is no small task, but if you start small, one step at a time, you will find the health benefits well worth it.

---

[21] Pacheco, D. 2023. "Alcohol and Sleep." Sleep Foundation (February 8). Retrieved February 14, 2023, from https://www.sleepfoundation.org/nutrition/alcohol-and-sleep.

Treating ourselves with kindness is a prerequisite for extending kindness to others.

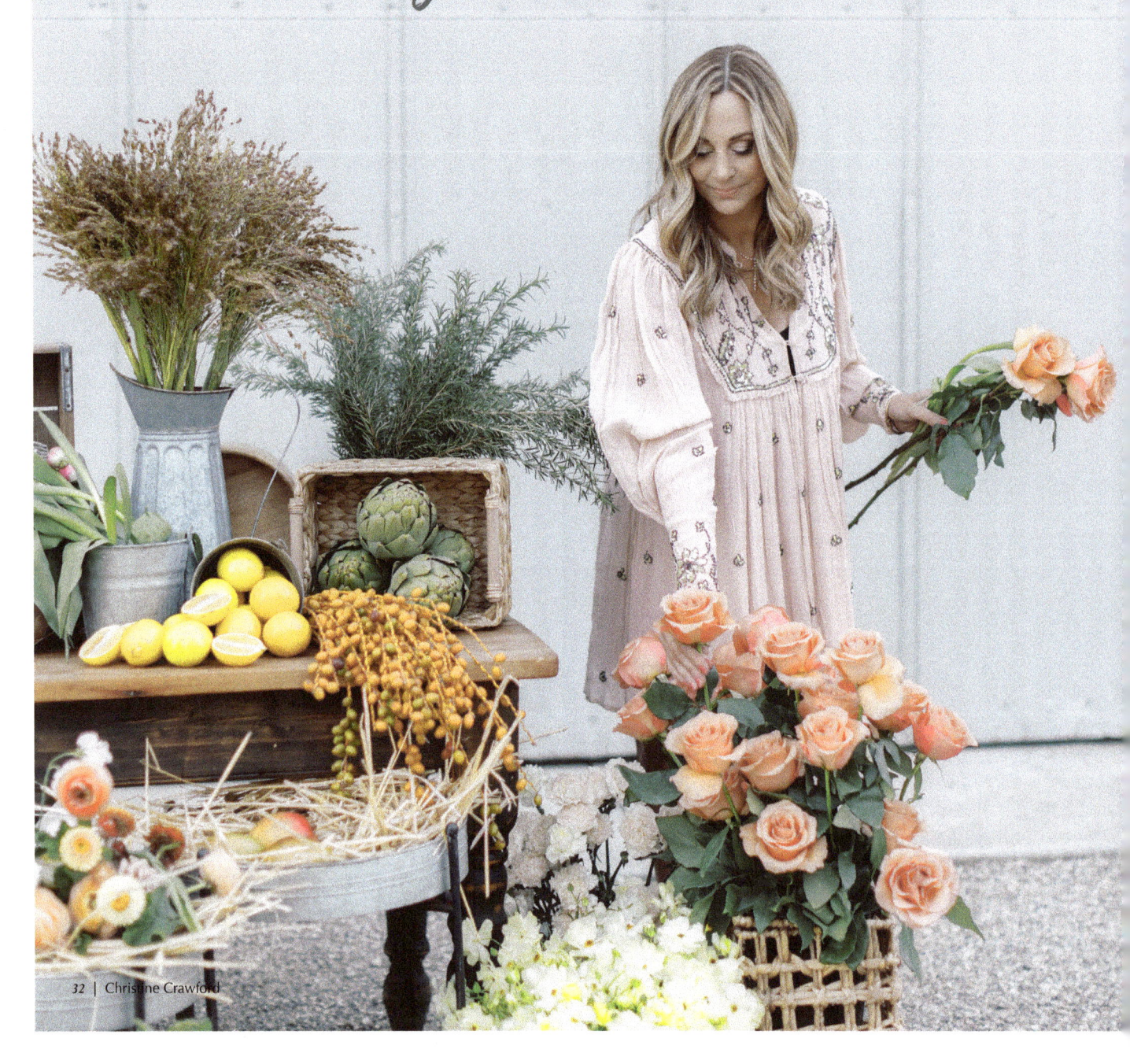

SOUL

We must find a special place in our hearts, minds, or nature—somewhere we can go every day, where there is no judgment or expectation, a place that wholly allows for the blossoming of our souls.

What is the soul?

Our soul is the spiritual or immaterial part of ourselves. It is the "little voice inside" urging us to become a better version of ourselves. It is the person that rises above our everyday egos to put the well-being of others ahead of our desires. It's the part of us that craves a connection with other beings and nature. Healthy relationships with ourselves and others are vital to maintaining a healthy soul.

Self-Love

"Self-love is an essential nutrient in our lives and is vital to nourishing our souls. We can nourish ourselves fully by practicing self-care and self-compassion. Self-love, rooted in knowing and nurturing internal strengths and grounded in personal values, is essential for growth, learning, and the fullness that comes with living your whole truth."
—*Megan Logan, MSW LCSW*

When we hear *self-love*, most think of massages, spa days, girls' nights out, and bubble baths. These are beautiful ways to honor ourselves, but they are not the most critical players in developing self-love.

In her book *Self Love Workbook for Women: Release Self-Doubt, Build Self-Compassion, and Embrace Who You Are,* Megan Logan writes about self-love and how we can achieve this often elusive goal.

As she explains, developing self-love is about honoring every aspect of our wellness and eliminating negative self-talk and destructive relationships. It's about creating a safe space for our emotions and following the path of our spirituality. It is a continuously unfolding journey that reveals more about who we are.[22]

Prioritizing self-love is imperative because when we don't, we spend our energy trying to please others, dashing about endlessly, measuring if we are good enough (performance reviews, numbers on a scale, test grades, likes on a post). But unfortunately, these measures never fulfill our need for love, as self-love is the only thing that will allow us to have real connections, reach our potential, and find peace.

Self-love involves developing an honest dialogue with ourselves. This allows us to discover our values and create a life free of self-destructive habits, filled with constructive choices that take us further along the journey toward our true selves. Self-love cultivates a kinder approach to the way we interact with ourselves. We start to talk to ourselves in a loving, supportive way. We become our own best friend who is encouraging and forgiving.

Loving ourselves allows us to share from our overflow. When our bucket is low on self-love, we can fall into unhealthy dependent, and needy relationships. When we love ourselves, we have healthier expectations of our relationships because we no longer look to others to fill the void and make us happy. It requires self-compassion, which is about releasing judgment of ourselves and treating ourselves with kindness.

Outlined in this book are numerous ways to love ourselves more. Still, if you want to delve deeper into a self-love journey, I recommend getting the book *Love Yourself Like Your Life Depends on It*, the expanded 2020 version by Kamal Ravikant, www.kamal.blog, *Self-Compassion, the Proven Power of Being Kind to Yourself,* by Kristin Neff, Ph.D., www.self-compassion.org. And specifically for women, *Self-Love Workbook for Women: Release Self-Doubt, Build Self-Compassion and Embrace Who You Are* by Megan Logan, MSW, LCSW. www.meganloganlcsw.com

---

22 Logan, M. (2020). *Self-Love Workbook for Women: Release Self-Doubt, Build Self-Compassion, and Embrace Who You Are.* New York: Rockridge Press.

Self-Compassion

Self-Compassion is treating ourselves with kindness and care as we would treat a dear friend. Many of us have learned the importance of treating our friends with kindness, especially when they have a tough time (e.g., making a big mistake at work). However, not all of us have learned how to treat ourselves similarly.

Imagine conversing with a friend who has just been through a breakup with their significant other. Imagine what you would say to them. Most likely, you wouldn't respond by telling them that it serves them right since they don't take care of themselves and are lazy, fat, and unattractive. But this is the way we often talk to ourselves. When we have self-compassion, we speak to ourselves the way we talk to a good friend. "Oh, honey, I'm sorry." "He doesn't know what he's lost."

Dr. Kristen Neff received her doctorate from the University of California at Berkeley and is a leading psychologist and self-compassion expert. Her book *Self-Compassion* explains that "self-compassion is a powerful way to achieve emotional well-being and contentment in our lives. By giving ourselves unconditional kindness and comfort while embracing the human experience, we avoid destructive patterns of fear, negativity, and isolation. At the same time, self-compassion fosters positive mind-states such as happiness and optimism."[23]

You can determine your precise level of self-compassion using the self-compassion scale developed by Kristen Neff for her research. Go to her website—and fill out the "Self-Compassionate Test". www.self-compassion.org/self-compassion-test. After filling out a series of questions, your level of self-compassion will be calculated for you.[24]

Self-esteem and self-compassion are different things. Self-esteem is how highly you value yourself based on accomplishments and comparison to others. Self-compassion acknowledges your flaws and limitations, allowing you to love and accept yourself as you are. We are imperfect and cannot always have high self-esteem, but we can always have self-compassion, like best friends walking through this life together.

Releasing Self-Doubt

When working to create self-love, we must examine and let go of negative thoughts and beliefs about ourselves. Sometimes our worst enemy comes in our self-sabotaging thought

---

23 Neff, Kristin. 2015. *Self-Compassion.* New York: HarperCollins, pp. 12–13. Kindle Edition.

24 Neff, K., and C. Germer. 2018. *The Mindful Self-Compassion Workbook: A Proven Way to Accept Yourself, Build Inner Strength, and Thrive.* New York: Guilford Press.

patterns. To build self-worth, we have to first find and eliminate sources of self-doubt and release limiting beliefs from our early childhood to the present. Some examples are "I'm an idiot," "I'm inadequate," and "I'm so lazy."

Everyone experiences limiting beliefs. We need not feel that our imperfections separate us from others; we probably share them with half a billion people. Most people experience periods of self-doubt and feelings of isolation.

The first thing to do is look at our negative core beliefs. Once we do this, we start to diminish their power. Then we need to notice our strengths. Everyone has both strengths and weaknesses. We must embrace all parts of ourselves.

By acknowledging our weaknesses with kindness, remembering that we are not alone in them, and recognizing our negative emotions related to them ("I feel bad") rather than identifying with them ("I am bad"), we release the shame and become whole again.[25]

Having self-limiting thoughts is natural, but that doesn't mean we need to listen to them. Below is a self-love and positive belief-building exercise.

To get started releasing self-doubt,

1. Identify and list your negative core beliefs. Here are some examples: "I am stupid, I am helpless, I am incapable, I am worthless."
2. Then notice if there are specific contexts in which they arise. Then write about what it feels like to hold these negative beliefs (e.g., "It hurts when I think I'm unloveable").
3. Then note where there is common human experience in this belief. For example, "I know so many people feel this same way. I am not alone."
4. Then write some words of kindness and understanding to yourself (e.g., "I'm sorry you feel this way. But please know that I love you and am here for you").[26]

Building Self-Worth

Working toward building self-worth is a journey. Below are some steps to get you started.

1. The first and most important step in loving ourselves is deciding to. You may call it a vow or anything you like, but we need to decide with an intention to love ourselves and do what we must do to make that happen.

---

25 Neff, K., and C. Germer. 2018. *The Mindful Self-Compassion Workbook: A Proven Way to Accept Yourself, Build Inner Strength, and Thrive*. New York: Guilford Press.

26 Neff, K., and C. Germer. 2018. *The Mindful Self-Compassion Workbook: A Proven Way to Accept Yourself, Build Inner Strength, and Thrive*. New York: Guilford Press, p. 125.

2. Recognize where a lack of self-love shows up in your life. Often, a lack of self-love reveals itself as a search for approval and attention from outside sources, which inevitably leaves us feeling more alone and empty inside. Keep a journal going and create an area for this. When you notice a lack of self-love, jot it down in your phone notes or whatever you have handy. Later, add them to your journal.
3. Set your intentions for what you want from your self-love journey.
    a. Ask yourself what you would like from this journey. Some examples include: I will be kinder to my body, I will have inner peace, I will develop more confidence, I will have better relationships.
    b. Jot down your answers, and then make a list in your journal.
4. Develop a daily self-love practice, which creates a direction and focus in our subconscious through affirmations.
    - Affirmations facilitate the reprogramming of the subconscious mind. According to Walter E. Jacobson, MD, our subconscious mind plays a significant role in actualizing our lives and manifesting our dreams. What we believe subconsciously, he says, can have a considerable impact on the outcome of events. Affirmations, repeated enough, reprogram old and faulty beliefs.[27] Affirmations are extremely useful in helping us create the lives we seek (e.g., attracting happiness, wealth, and love and training our brains to think kind and positive thoughts about ourselves). With repetition and buy-in, we cement beliefs in our subconscious minds. We must feel the emotions we would have as if the affirmation is already true. For example, "I am worthy of love." Imagine how you would feel if this was true. Step into the feeling, embrace it, let it encompass your whole body, and revel in it. Your subconscious mind needs proof. Feeling emotions is a way to give it the evidence it needs.

        Here are some examples. Try writing some of your own.
    - I am comfortable in my body.
    - I am worthy of love.
    - I deserve happiness and joy.
    - I trust my intuition.
    - My feelings are valid.
    - Loving myself is important.
    - Journaling work: In your journal, list any negative beliefs or labels given to you by yourself or others. For example, "I am such a loser," "I always mess everything up," and "I am fat and ugly." Next, I would like you to write a positive belief or

---

27 Lively, K. J. 2014. "Affirmations: The Why, What, How, and What If?" *Psychology Today* (March 12). Retrieved February 14, 2023, from https://www.psychologytoday.com/us/blog/smart-relationships/201403/affirmations-the-why-what-how-and-what-if.

label beside each negative one. For example, "I am a winner," "I am capable," and "I am attractive."

- Imagery work: The brain learns through images and symbols, making them essential for communicating with our minds. Using imagery, we use words to evoke imaginary scenarios bringing many benefits.

"Imagery, including forms of rescripting—the imagined change of the course of events in memories or fantasies of aversive experiences—has been used as a therapeutic technique for over 20,000 years."[28]

Visualization and guided imagery connect the brain's visual cortex and the involuntary nervous system to bring therapeutic benefits.

This imagery exercise is something I developed for use with my clients. Try it for yourself:

1. Find a place where you are comfortable and free from distractions—where you can focus on deep relaxation.
2. Get into a comfortable position, sitting or lying down. Uncross your arms and legs.
3. Take three slow deep breaths, fully exhaling until your lungs are empty, and close your eyes.
4. Imagine standing in front of a whiteboard. All the beliefs and labels from the journaling exercise above are on it.
5. Take an eraser from the ledge and erase the first belief or label. Then move down the list, erasing each.
6. Tell yourself that these no longer have any power over you as you are erasing.
7. After you have erased all the negative words, take a new marker from the box on the ledge.
8. Begin writing the positive beliefs and labels.
9. After you have written all of them, step back and stand before the board. Take a moment to feel the energy of each one and connect with the emotion of gratitude for the unique and beautiful person you are.
10. Smile from deep in your soul, knowing that no one is quite like you, that you are unique, special, and loved.
11. Take a few moments to marinate in these feelings.
12. Now, slowly begin to wake. Wiggle your fingers and toes. Open your eyes.

---

28 Arntz, A. 2011. "Imagery Rescripting as a Therapeutic Technique: Review of Clinical Trials, Basic Studies, and Research Agenda." *Journal of Experimental Psychopathology* 3 (2): 189–208. Retrieved February 15, 2023, from https://journals.sagepub.com/doi/pdf/10.5127/jep.024211.

Learning to love ourselves is a continuous journey. It involves deliberate effort and practice. It also requires honesty, courage, and vulnerability. It does not mean we are perfect, but rather that we are working toward finding our authentic selves through self-compassion and kindness. Do these steps before bed because when we are about to sleep, our minds drift into hypnosis, opening our subconscious.

Some other ways to show yourself love throughout the day are:

- Get a positive affirmations app for your phone. I love the "I Am" app. You can customize it according to your preferences. There are categories such as Confidence, Self-Love, Health and Well-being, Positive Thinking, and many more. You choose how many reminders you would like to see in a day. I set mine to fifteen daily reminders between 8:00 a.m. and 10:00 p.m. My messages include affirmations such as:
  - I will give myself the love and patience I give others.
  - I am proud of myself for getting this far.
  - I accept myself as I am and love whom I am becoming.
  - I am worthy of true love.
- Write a letter describing your highest self. Here is mine:

    I am love and light, and I savor a profound connection to the present. I am compassionate, kind, and loving, and need validation only from myself. My gaze is upward, toward the sun, and I am always moving forward. I give to those in need and receive in kind. I am a shining example of self-love and mastery, and inspire others to see themselves through my eyes. I have wealth and abundance and am fully immersed in this life on our beautiful planet. I radiate beauty from deep within, and it illuminates the world around me. I am an inspiration for all, and I fully trust God and the universe and their divine timing.

Relationships

When the study began, nobody cared about empathy or attachment.
But the key to healthy aging is relationships, relationships, relationships.
—George Vaillant

In 1938, Harvard scientists began one of the world's most extensive studies of adult human life. The Grant and Glueck study began tracking 268 Harvard sophomores during the Great Depression. They hoped the study would give insight into living a happy, healthy life.

They were not disappointed!

After following the original 268 students for nearly 80 years, they added 456 Boston residents in the 1970s and 10 years ago added the wives of the original students. They collected a bevy of data on physical and mental health.

Robert Waldinger is the director of the study and professor of psychiatry at Harvard Medical School. The most surprising information he found from the study results is that happiness in our relationships extensively influences our health.

He said, "Taking care of your body is important, but tending to your relationships is a form of self-care too. That, I think, is the revelation."[29]

In 1966, psychiatrist George Vaillant joined the team and led the study until 2004. Vaillant highlighted the role of relationships and stressed their importance in achieving long and happy lives.

We now know of an established way to improve our lives. So how do we cultivate good relationships? It is a fundamental cornerstone of our lives but sometimes seems like a forgotten art.

---

29 Mineo, L. 2018. "Over Nearly 80 Years, Harvard Study Has Been Showing How to Live a Healthy and Happy Life." *Harvard Gazette* (November 26). Retrieved February 15, 2023, from https://news.harvard.edu/gazette/story/2017/04/over-nearly-80-years-harvard-study-has-been-showing-how-to-live-a-healthy-and-happy-life/.

Trust

Trust is paramount to building a good relationship, and it is imperative if we want love to last.

"Our partner should be our respite from the outside world, a soft spot for us to land. For trust to exist and grow, we need to know that our partner 'gets us,' has our best interests, and that we can depend on them to be available, i.e., be physically and emotionally present for us," says Jessica L. Griffin, associate professor of psychiatry and pediatrics at the University of Massachusetts Medical School in Worcester.[30]

To build trust, we need to embody:

- Sincerity—Sincerity builds trust. The word means "free from pretense or deceit; proceeding from genuine feelings." We develop sincerity daily by being genuine in interacting with our partners, friends, and colleagues. When we are sincere, we are believable. Even minor inconsistencies, if habitual, signal to your partner that they should not trust what you say and do.
- Respect—Andrea Bonior, PhD, of *Psychology Today*, said, "One of the most emotionally lasting ways our partners can damage us—and our trust—is by belittling us, making us feel less-than, or viewing us with condescension or contempt rather than respect."[31] Respect means to regard. It is about respecting someone the way they are and holding their feelings, emotions, and beliefs with the same value that we hold our own, even though we might not share them. Respect builds trust and feelings of safety and well-being in relationships. Respect does not always come naturally, but we can learn it.

For those who have experienced instability, harm, or alienation in their early years, lack of trust can manifest as avoidance of intimacy and isolation. But, like most good things, trust must be worked on and maintained.

---

[30] Courtney, N. J. 2021. "Trust in a Relationship: Why It's Important and How to Build It." The Healthy (April 2). Retrieved February 15, 2023, from https://www.thehealthy.com/family/relationships/trust-in-a-relationship/

[31] Bonlor, Andrea. 2018. "7 Ways to Build Trust in a Relationship." Psychology Today (December 12). https://www.psychologytoday.com/us/blog/friendship-20/201812/7-ways-build-trust-in-relationship.

Communication in Relationships

Effective communication is essential for fostering and maintaining a healthy connection in any personal or professional partnership. Through communication, individuals express their thoughts, emotions, and needs. The absence of effective communication can lead to feelings of disconnection, misunderstanding, or lack of support, resulting in isolation and discontent.

Effective communication nurtures close emotional ties and intimacy, strengthens trust and respect, and improves collaborative problem-solving. It plays a crucial role in allowing individuals to better appreciate each other's viewpoints and needs.

Signs that you may have communication problems in a relationship:

- Blaming
- Assuming
- Arguing frequently
- Resentment
- Defensiveness
- Decreased affection
- No Communication - shutting down
- Criticizing
- Lying
- Stubbornness
- Aggressiveness
- Passive-aggressiveness
- Distrust
- Jealousy

Common Communication Challenges in Relationships

Lack of active listening

Active listening is fundamental to successful communication. It requires fully concentrating on our partners' words, observing their tone, body language, and emotions, and responding in a way that shows consideration and appreciation for their needs, worries, and importance to us.

We can achieve active listening when we
- Focus on what our partner says, keep eye contact, and refrain from interrupting,
- Ask open-ended questions that encourage responses,
- Listen to understand, not to respond,
- Pay attention to non-verbal cues,
- Repeat back what has been said,
- Withhold advice and judgment.[32]

Lack of Empathy

Empathy involves recognizing and connecting with our partner's feelings and experiences. It's an essential element of successful communication. We can do this by stepping into our partner's shoes and comprehending their feelings. This approach helps us better understand their viewpoint, enabling us to respond in a compassionate and supportive way.

Using You Statements

When we use "you" statements, we can make our partner feel shame or blame, potentially resulting in defensiveness and animosity. This can make it challenging to resolve conflicts and communicate effectively. Instead, we can use statements such as "I feel," "I want," or "I need," which allows us to convey our emotions and needs without casting blame or attacking our partner. This approach can foster a sense of being heard and understood, contributing to more productive communication.

Difficulty Compromising

Compromise plays a vital role in healthy communication, as it involves identifying solutions that accommodate the needs and desires of both partners. Sadly, many people in relationships find compromise challenging, which often leads to power struggles and conflicts.

Claudia de Llano, LMFT, a licensed marriage and family therapist and author of "The Seven Destinies of Love" says "Compromise entails a mutual respect and regard for each other's feelings and needs. "It is an invitation to collaborate with your partner while solving problems".

In a relationship, it's common for partners to hold different values, tastes, or habits. You might, for example, disagree on which movie to watch or vacation destination. These kinds of differences can spark conflicts, as each person may want something different, and there may not be a straightforward solution. This is where the importance of compromise becomes evident.

---

32 Cuncic, A., MA. (2024b, February 12). *7 Active listening techniques for better communication.* Verywell Mind. https://www.verywellmind.com/what-is-active-listening-3024343

The ability to compromise plays a crucial role in resolving disagreements. When either partner consistently refuses to find middle ground, insisting on their own way, it often results in frequent disputes. This pattern can gradually weaken the bond of the relationship.

Compromise in relationships involves both partners collaborating towards a mutual goal. This means relinquishing individual preferences to move forward in the relationship.

But it's important to distinguish between compromise and sacrifice. Sacrifice typically involves one partner yielding more than the other or acting alone to enhance the other's happiness. In contrast, mutual respect characterizes true compromise and equal contributions from both partners for the benefit of the relationship.

If you and your partner find communication challenging, it may be beneficial to seek guidance from a therapist or counselor. A professional can assist in pinpointing and tackling communication issues, offering the necessary tools and techniques to foster a healthier, more joyful relationship.

Intimacy

When we think of the word 'intimacy,' many of us think of sexual relations, but intimacy extends beyond physical closeness in romantic settings. It also includes the deep connection found in friendships and other non-romantic relationships. Intimacy can present emotionally, physically, sexually, spiritually, or platonically.

Some indicators of emotional intimacy with someone may include:

- They accept our flaws and do not pressure us to change.
- They keep our secrets confidential.
- They understand and empathize with our emotions. Even if they don't always agree with our choices, they continue to support us.
- They care for us and are willing to assist us whenever they can.

Intimacy, whether platonic or sexual can help us cope with stress, build positive experiences, and pursue our goals. Here are some non-sexual ways of including intimacy in our lives.

- Physical gestures: Holding, hugging, cuddling, kissing.
- Emotional support: Being present in a friend's life, listening to them, and providing emotional support.
- Vulnerability: Sharing emotional moments, or being transparent about your truth.

Spirituality

Spirituality…It feeds you more deeply than the food on your plate because it reminds you that you're connected to something larger than yourself.
—Institute for Integrative Nutrition[33]

Spirituality is abstract, ambiguous, and highly subjective. It is the experience of connecting with something larger than ourselves. It is the discovery of meaning and purpose in our lives. It has been defined as "experiencing transcendence through inner peace, harmony, or connectedness to others."[34]

Many of us take care of our minds and bodies. We exercise, eat healthy, set intentions, and see therapists, but at the end of the day, we still feel like something is missing. Some may feel tired and empty or ruminate endlessly about the past or future.

For many, spirituality may be the missing piece. I'm not talking about religion. Religion is a set of beliefs and practices shared with a group. For me, spirituality is highly individual. It is about connecting with the universe, nature, and humanity. A friend of mine who considers herself agnostic said that as she grows older, she experiences episodes where she begins to weep on her daily bike rides, not out of sadness but gratitude for the beauty she sees. I explained that she was experiencing spirituality. She was connecting with nature and was moved by it, whereas previously, she rode her bike with her air pods blasting music and didn't connect with her surroundings.

Maintaining a spiritual practice has been shown to calm anxiety, ease stress, improve mood, and more. In addition, many studies have shown that spirituality positively affects the quality of life. One such study, the American Cancer Society's Study of Cancer Survivors,

---

33 Rosenthal, J. 2021. "Is Spirituality the Key to Health?" Institute for Integrative Nutrition (March 4). Retrieved February 15, 2023, from https://www.integrativenutrition.com/blog/is-spirituality-the-key-to-health#:~:text=Spirituality%20is%20an%20important%20part,Reduces%20stress.

34 Boswell, G. H., E. Kahana, and P. Dilworth-Anderson. 2006. "Spirituality and Healthy Lifestyle Behaviors: Stress Counter-Balancing Effects on the Well-Being of Older Adults. Journal of Religion and Health (November 7). SpringerLink. Retrieved February 15, 2023, from https://link.springer.com/article/10.1007/s10943-006-9060-7.

found that spirituality was an independent predictor of a better quality of life and emotional well-being. A separate analysis of this data found that faith contributed significantly to cancer survivors' functional quality of life—nearly 70 percent of participants reported that spirituality helped them through their cancer experience.[35]

If you aren't experiencing spirituality in your life, here are some ways to tap into this vast pool of energy.

- Experiment with meditation or yoga stretching in a quiet environment.
- Get out in nature. Connecting with what we hear, feel, see, and smell can bring our consciousness to a higher plane.
- Spend time alone each day. It doesn't have to be for a long time. When we spend most of our time doing, doing, doing, we miss the being side of ourselves. Our inner selves crave connection. We feed our souls by connecting with ourselves, being still, and just sitting with ourselves.
- Serve others. When I'm disillusioned or empty, I ask myself, "What can I do for others?" Taking time to help another being, even if it's as small as taking the dogs for a walk, lifts our spirits. We become aware that our presence serves a higher purpose.
- Write a gratitude list or journal about the things you are grateful for. Starting or ending our days with gratitude is a powerful way to tune in to our spirituality.

Spirituality doesn't need to be complex. So take a few minutes today, do something for another person, or try some yoga. The amount of inner fulfillment will be well worth your time.

---

35 Canada, A. L., P. E. Murphy, G. Fitchett, and K. Stein. 2016. "Re-Examining the Contributions of Faith, Meaning, and Peace to Quality of Life: A Report from the American Cancer Society's Studies of Cancer Survivors- II (SCS-II)." Annals of Behavioral Medicine: A Publication of the Society of Behavioral Medicine 50 (1): 79–86. Retrieved February 15, 2023, from https://pubmed.ncbi.nlm.nih.gov/26384498/.

THE RECIPES

The recipes I've compiled here are low-energy-density (LED), filling foods. They are low in sugar, hydrating, high in protein and fiber, and are nutrient-dense. When choosing what to eat, consider how filling and nutrient dense a food is for its calorie content. LED foods lead to more fullness and satisfaction after eating, which can help manage hunger and reduce the likelihood of overeating.

LED foods often have a higher nutritional value. They are typically rich in essential nutrients like vitamins, minerals, and antioxidants. This aspect of the diet can lead to better overall health and well-being.

Unlike restrictive diets, a LED diet can be more sustainable and easier to adhere to in the long term. It allows for a larger volume of food to be consumed, which can make it more satisfying and less restrictive. For those wanting to manage our weight, studies show LED meals improve appetite control, and the effect is sustainable.[36]

Rather than cutting out foods we like, such as those high in fat and carbohydrate content, try consuming a large volume of LED food, such as soup, salad, or fruit, as a first course to boost satiety, increase nutrient content and reduce overall calorie intake at a meal.

36 Buckland NJ, Camidge D, Croden F, Lavin JH, Stubbs RJ, Hetherington MM, Blundell JE, Finlayson G. A Low Energy-Dense Diet in the Context of a Weight-Management Program Affects Appetite Control in Overweight and Obese Women. J Nutr. 2018 May 1;148(5):798-806. doi: 10.1093/jn/nxy041. PMID: 30053284; PMCID: PMC6054218.

BOWLS

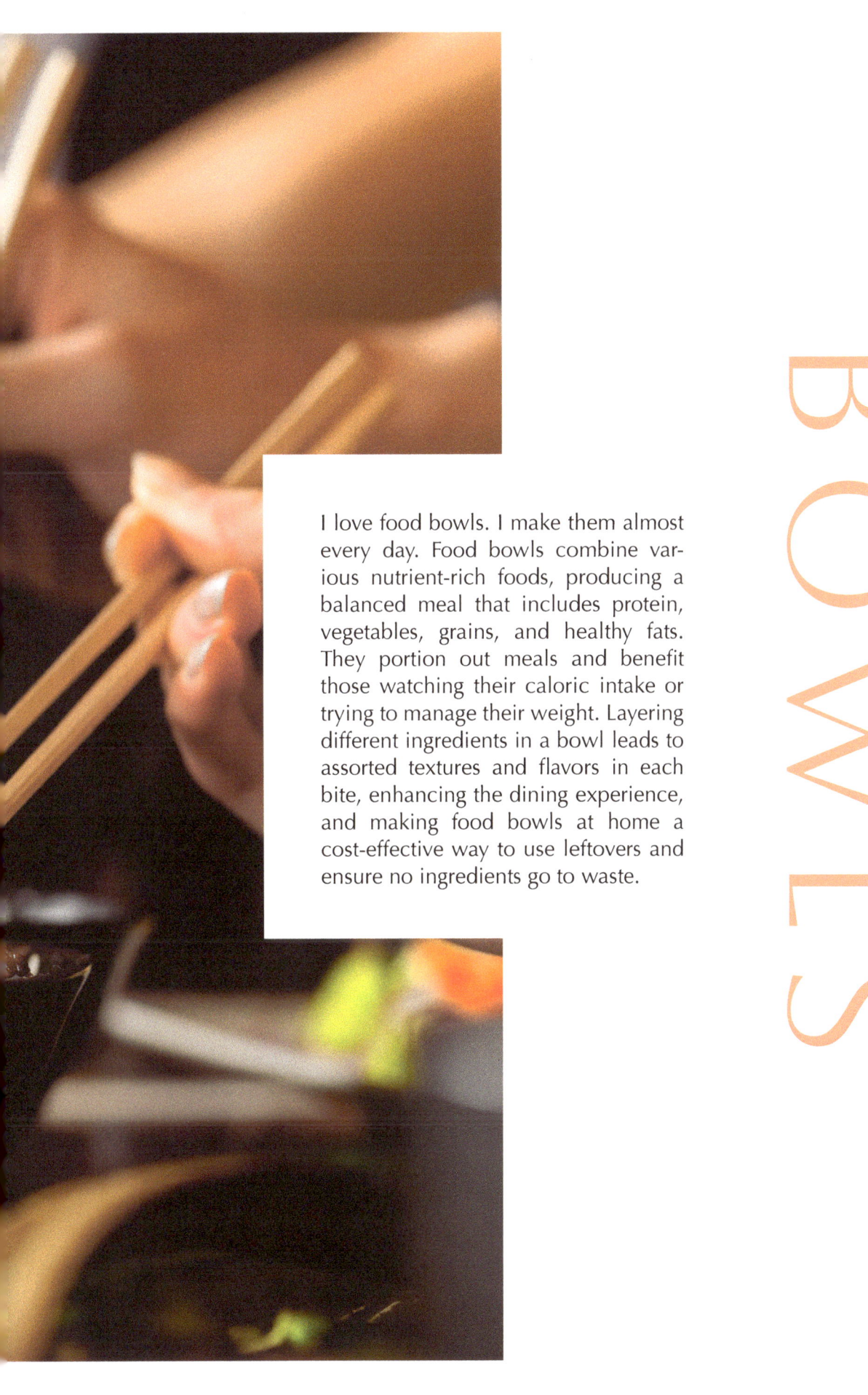

I love food bowls. I make them almost every day. Food bowls combine various nutrient-rich foods, producing a balanced meal that includes protein, vegetables, grains, and healthy fats. They portion out meals and benefit those watching their caloric intake or trying to manage their weight. Layering different ingredients in a bowl leads to assorted textures and flavors in each bite, enhancing the dining experience, and making food bowls at home a cost-effective way to use leftovers and ensure no ingredients go to waste.

DRAGON FRUIT (PITAYA) SMOOTHIE BOWL

Dragon fruit, also known as pitaya or pitahaya, gives a vibrant color to your smoothie bowl and provides a range of health benefits. Here's a simple and delicious recipe for a dragon fruit smoothie bowl:

PREP TIME 10 minutes, BLEND AND SERVE 5 minutes
TOTAL TIME 15 minutes, SERVINGS 1 bowl

INGREDIENTS

- 1 ripe dragon fruit either white or red-fleshed
- 1 frozen banana sliced
- 1/2 cup frozen mixed berries like blueberries, raspberries, or strawberries
- 1/2 cup unsweetened almond milk or coconut milk, or any milk of your choice
- 1 tbsp. chia seeds optional for added texture and nutrients
- granola fresh berries, sliced kiwi, coconut flakes, chia seeds, nuts, or any of your favorite toppings

INSTRUCTIONS

1. Slice the dragon fruit in half. Use a spoon to scoop out the flesh from one half and set aside the other half to use as a serving bowl (optional).

2. In a blender, combine the dragon fruit flesh, frozen banana slices, frozen berries, coconut milk, and chia seeds (if using). Blend until smooth. If the mixture is too thick, add more milk to achieve your desired consistency.

3. Pour the smoothie mixture into a bowl (or the scooped-out dragon fruit skin for a more natural and eye-catching presentation).

4. Decorate with your choice of toppings. Granola adds a nice crunch, berries provide freshness, coconut flakes offer tropical flair, and nuts add texture and protein.

5. Enjoy immediately!

NOTES

You can customize this smoothie bowl by adding protein powder, different fruits, or yogurt to change the texture and flavor.

Nurturing Mind, Body, and Soul | 51

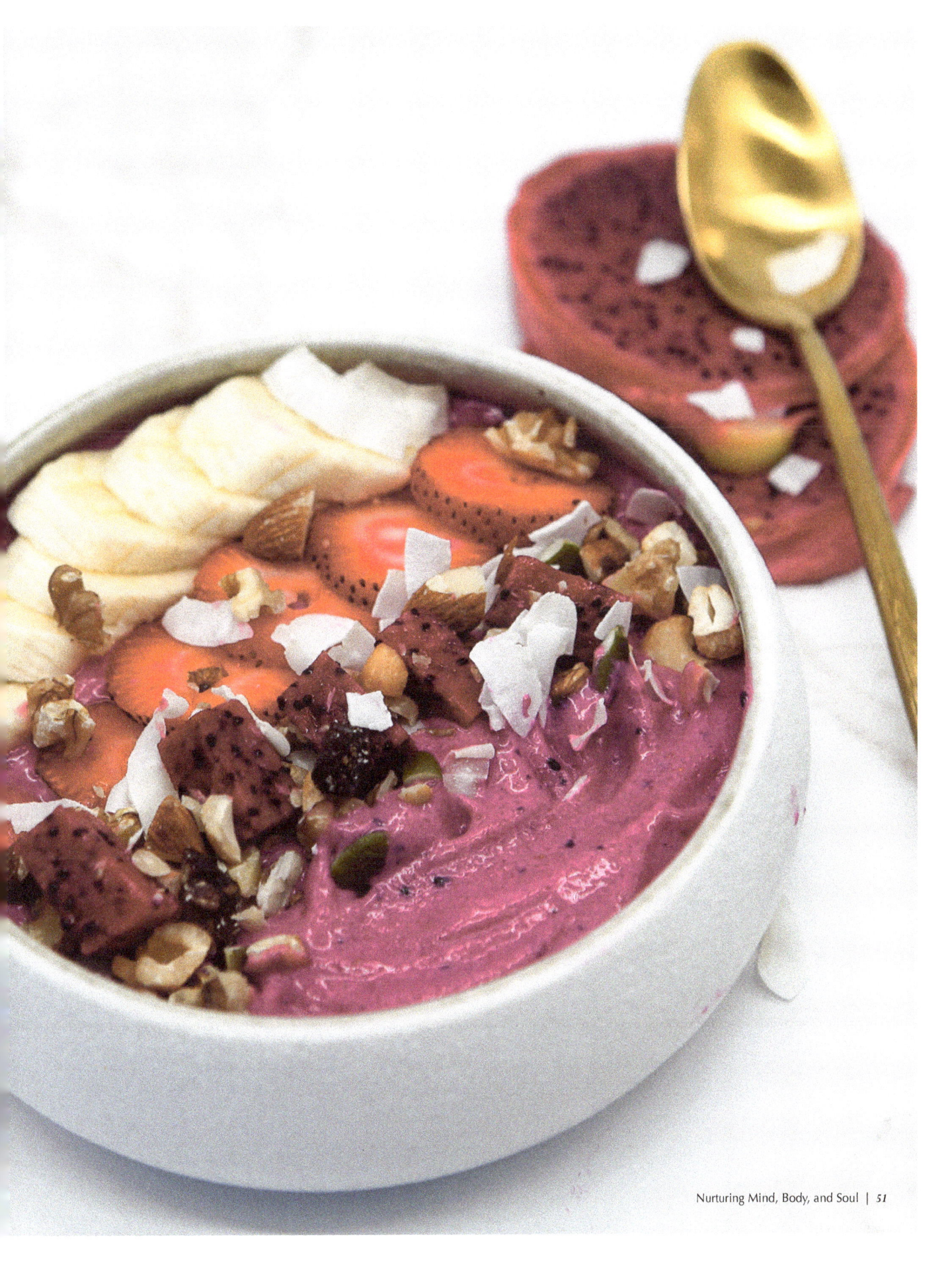

SPRING ROLL BOWL

These Spring Roll Bowls have bright, colorful ingredients. According to the food pyramid, we should consume up to nine servings of vegetables and fruits each day. You can eat a rainbow of colors with this satisfying, tasty bowl!

PREP TIME 30 minutes, TOTAL TIME 30 minutes, SERVINGS 2 bowls

INGREDIENTS

- 8 oz. rice noodles I like Thai Kitchens Stir-fry Rice Noodles
- 1 bell pepper washed sliced into thin strips
- 1/2 avocado sliced
- 1/2 zucchini spiralized
- 1 carrot sliced into thin strips
- 1/4 head purple cabbage sliced into thin strips
- 1 lime washed and cut into wedges
- sriracha to taste
- basil washed and torn as optional garnish

Sweet Soy Sauce
- 1 tsp. fresh garlic
- 1/4 cup fresh lime juice
- 2 tbsp. orange juice
- 1/4 cup soy sauce
- 1/4 cup sesame tahini
- 1 tsp. sriracha (optional)
- 1/2 cup neutral-tasting oil such as grapeseed oil or avocado oil

Garnish
- 1 or 2 leaves basil chiffonade
- 1 tsp. crushed red pepper
- 1/4 cup cashews chopped

INSTRUCTIONS

1. Cook the rice noodles per the package directions but add some neutral-flavored oil to the pot. When done, rinse the noodles with cold water to stop cooking. Drain the noodles and immediately toss them with 1/2 cup of neutral-flavored oil to prevent clumping.

2. In a small food processor, prepare the sweet soy sauce by combining the garlic, fresh lime juice, soy sauce, sugar, tahini, and Sriracha. Stir in the neutral-flavored oil.

3. Add the desired amount of Sweet Soy Sauce to the noodles and toss to coat.

4. Prepare each serving bowl with the noodle salad. Add the purple cabbage, bell pepper, zucchini, carrots, and avocado to the bowl with the rice noodles. Top with the sliced avocado and lime wedges. Garnish with chopped cashews, crushed red pepper, micro cilantro, and sweet soy sauce.

NOTES: Want to add a protein to your spring roll bowls? Steamed shrimp is a great option!

Nurturing Mind, Body, and Soul | 53

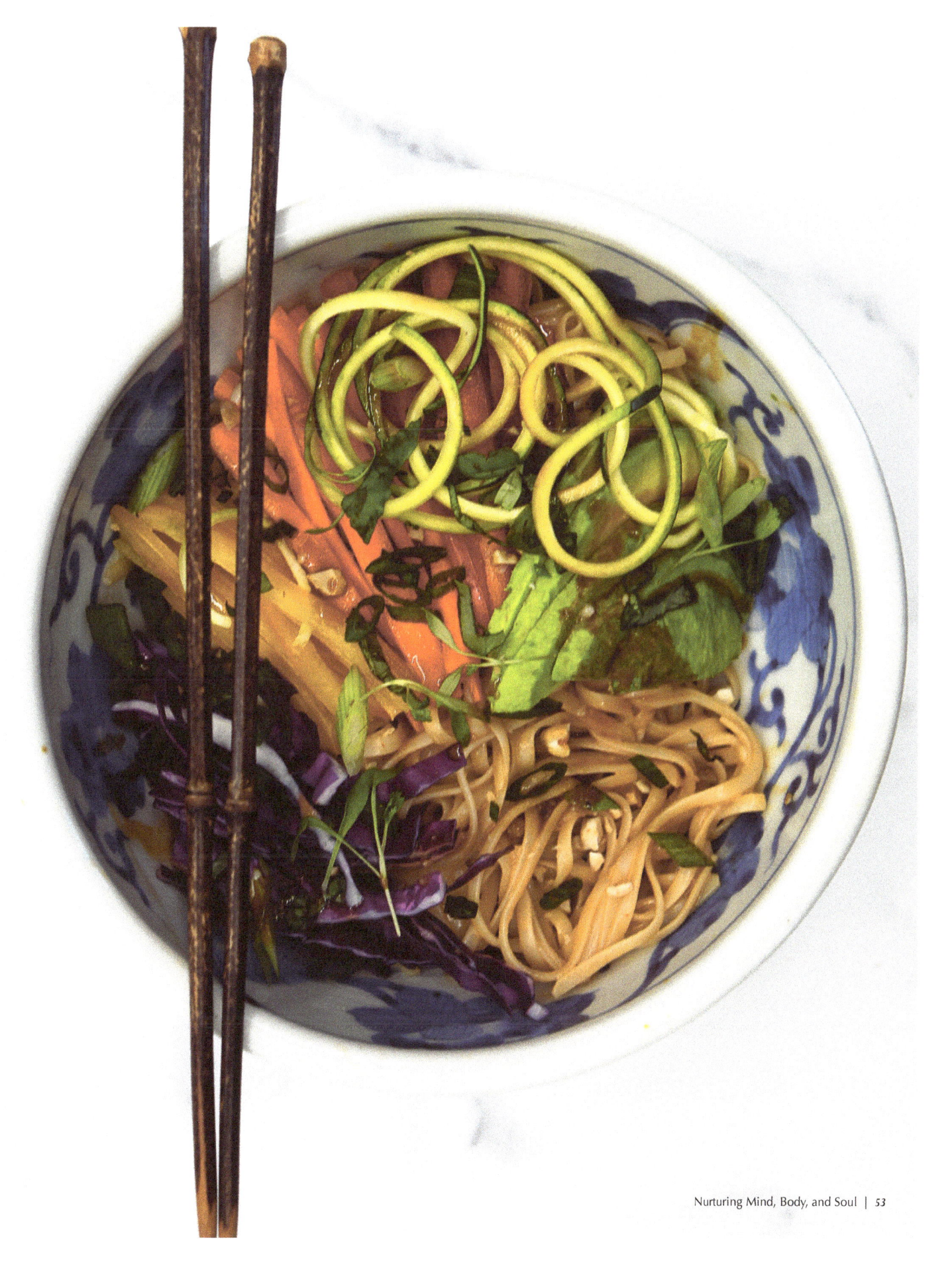

SPICY HAWAIIAN SALMON BOWL

This recipe will give your salmon a delightful balance of sweet, savory, spicy, and aromatic notes. Packed full of healthy fat, and loads of flavor, this one is a staple!

PREP TIME 10 minutes, COOK TIME 8 minutes, RESTING TIME 5 minutes, TOTAL TIME 23 minutes, SERVINGS 2 bowls

INGREDIENTS

- 2 lbs. salmon fillets or center-cut
- 1 tbsp. garlic powder
- 1 tsp. ginger powder
- 1 tbsp. paprika sweet or smoked: 1 tbsp.
- 1 tsp. cayenne powder adjust based on your heat preference
- Zest of 1 lime
- 1 tsp. dried cilantro optional
- 1 tbsp. sesame seeds optional
- 3 tbsp. Soy Sauce

For Spicy Mayo
- 3 tbsp. mayonnaise
- 1 tbsp. sriracha sauce

Toppings
- 3 stalks scallions
- 1 tbsp. sesame seeds

INSTRUCTIONS

1. In a bowl, mix all the dry ingredients thoroughly.
2. Brush soy sauce onto the salmon cubes
3. Coat cubes thoroughly with the dry spice mix.
4. Let the salmon marinate with the rub for 15-30 minutes in the refrigerator for the flavors to meld.
5. Preheat your broiler and arrange the salmon cubes on a sheet pan with foil.
6. Broil for about 8-15 minutes, or until the salmon is cooked through and the exterior is slightly caramelized, keeping an eye on it to prevent burning.
7. Combine mayonnaise and Sriracha to suit your taste.
8. Arrange salmon morsels on top of rice, and top with the Sriracha mayo, sesame seeds, and chopped scallions.
9. Enjoy!

Nurturing Mind, Body, and Soul | 55

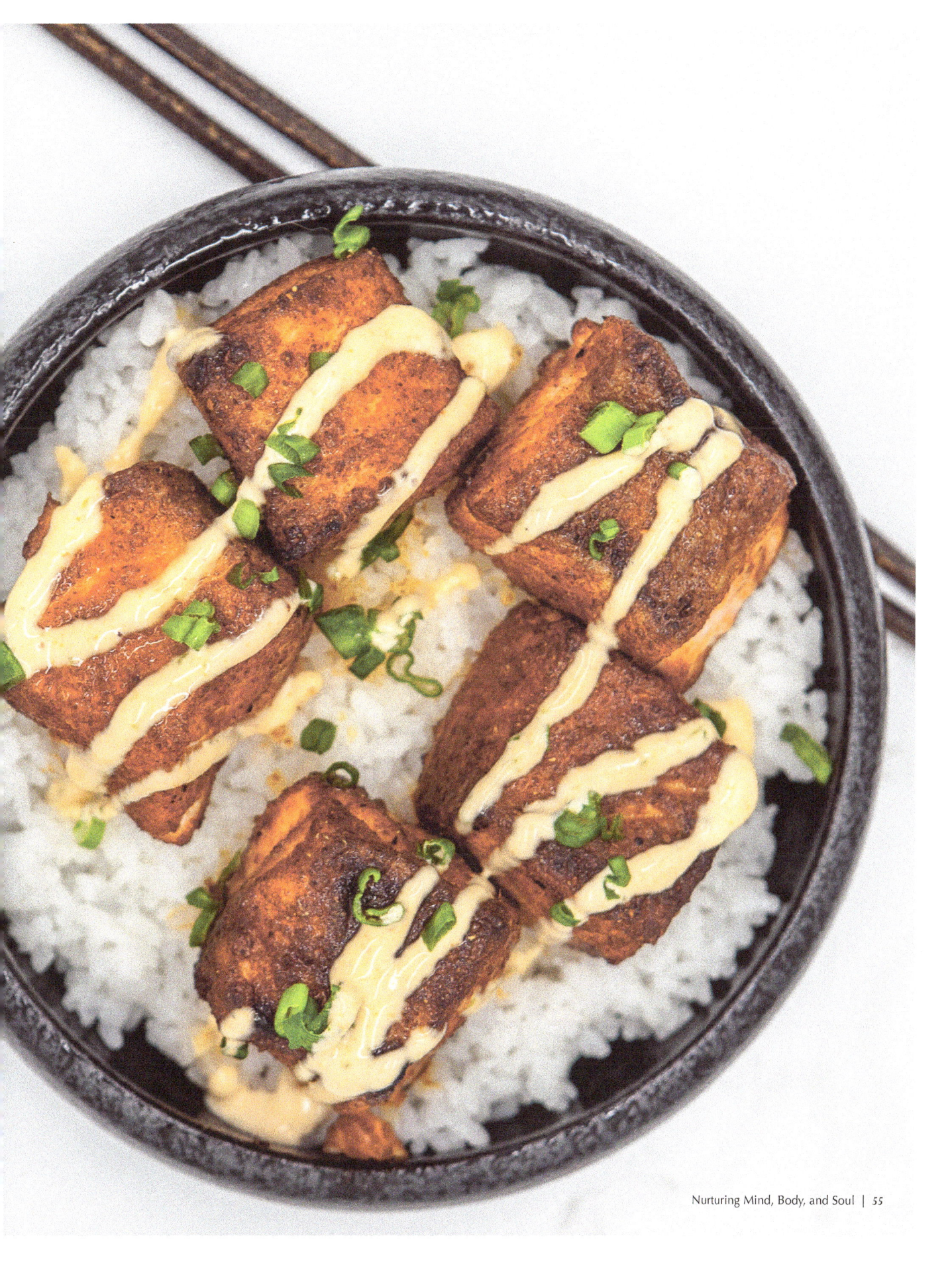

56 | Christine Crawford

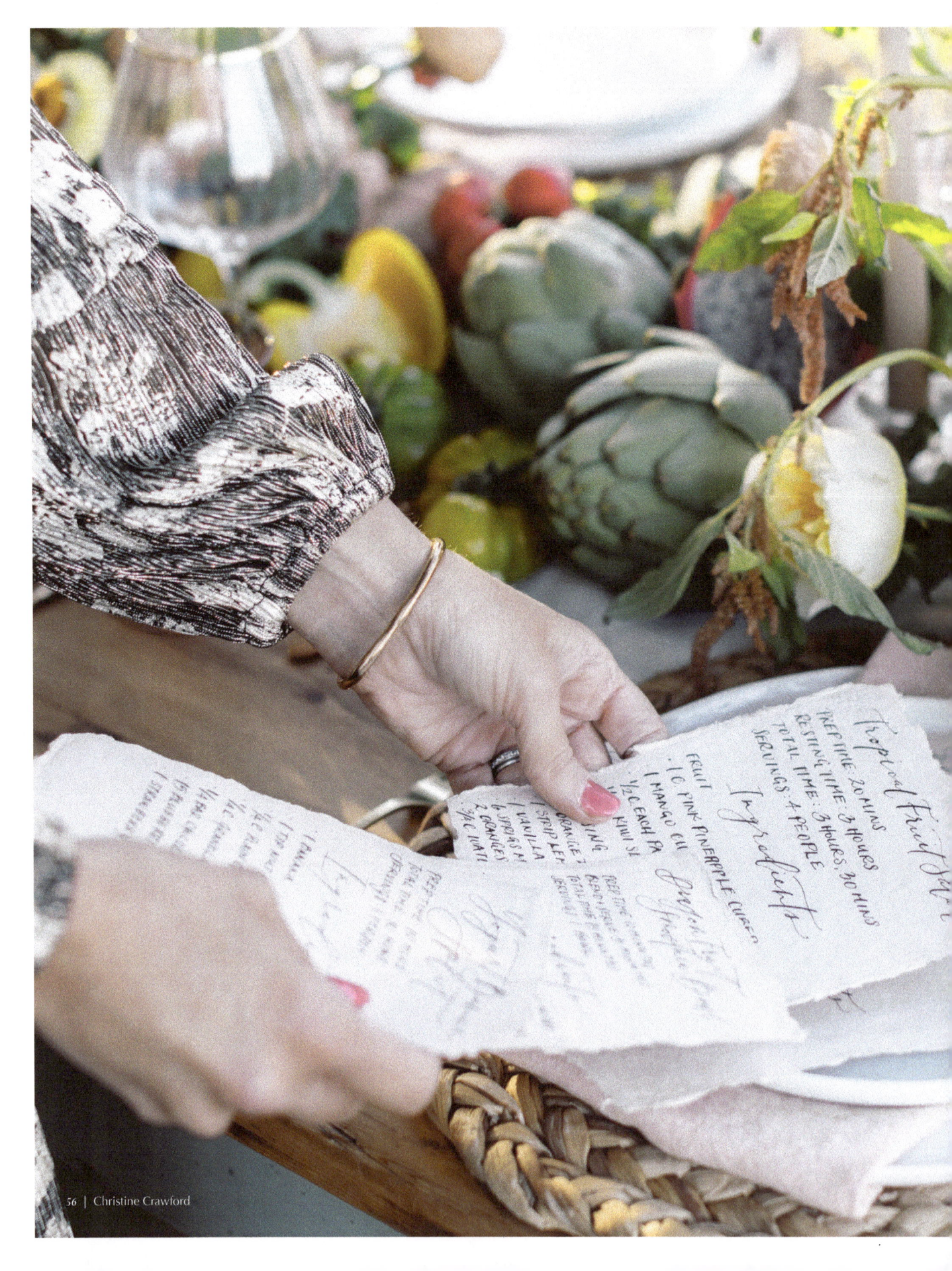

SALADS, SOUP, AND MORE

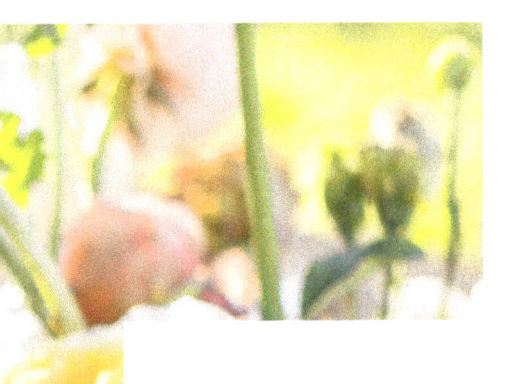

The following dishes employ different colors and textures, and include low-energy-density foods.

Adding color and texture to our meals isn't just a feast for the eyes; it's great for our health too! Vividly colored fruits and vegetables are packed with a wide array of vitamins, minerals, and antioxidants. Each color represents different nutrients.

For instance, red produce often contains lycopene, while green veggies are rich in chlorophyll. This rainbow of nutrients supports various bodily functions, from boosting your immune system to reducing inflammation.

Texture also plays a crucial role. Foods with varied textures encourage slower eating and can enhance the satisfaction and enjoyment of a meal. Crunchy vegetables, chewy grains, and creamy yogurts each require different chewing times and effort, which can help improve digestion and satiety. In essence, incorporating various colors and textures into your diet is a delightful and effective way to nurture your body and keep it functioning at its best.

TROPICAL FRUIT SALAD
(NO ADDED SUGAR)

This fresh and hydrating Tropical Fruit Salad is easier to achieve than you might think. I found pink pineapple and dragon fruit (pitaya) at my local grocery store. These days, we can get most any ingredients we want. I like to make something like this occasionally to mix up the fruit in my diet. If you haven't tried dragon fruit, I highly recommend it. This is an easy and delicious salad that will surprise your family and friends.

PREP TIME 20 minutes, RESTING TIME 3 hours
TOTAL TIME 3 hours 30 minutes, SERVINGS 4 people

INGREDIENTS

Fruit

- 1 cup pink pineapple cubed. I get this at my local grocery.
- 1 mango cubed. I get this at my local grocery.
- 1/2 cup papaya cubed. I get this at my local grocery.
- 1/2 cup dragon fruit cubed. This is also available at my local grocer.
- 1/2 cup kiwi sliced

Dressing

- 1 orange zest in strips
- 1 strip lemon zest
- 1 vanilla bean split
- 6 sprigs mint
- 2 oranges juiced
- 3/4 cup water

INSTRUCTIONS

1. Cut up pineapple, mango, dragon fruit, and kiwi.
2. Scrape any pith (the white part) off the zest strips and discard. Combine the orange and lemon zest, vanilla bean, mint, orange juice, and water in a saucepan. Bring to a boil. Turn to low and let simmer for 15 minutes or until you have 1/2 cup of liquid. Remove from the heat and let stand for at least 2 hours. Strain.
3. Stir the fruit into the syrup and refrigerate for an hour. Garnish with a mint sprig.

NOTES: You can eat this salad as is or use it as a topping for granola, yogurt, or smoothie bowls. You could enjoy it with ice cream or serve it with grilled chicken or fish.

Nurturing Mind, Body, and Soul | 59

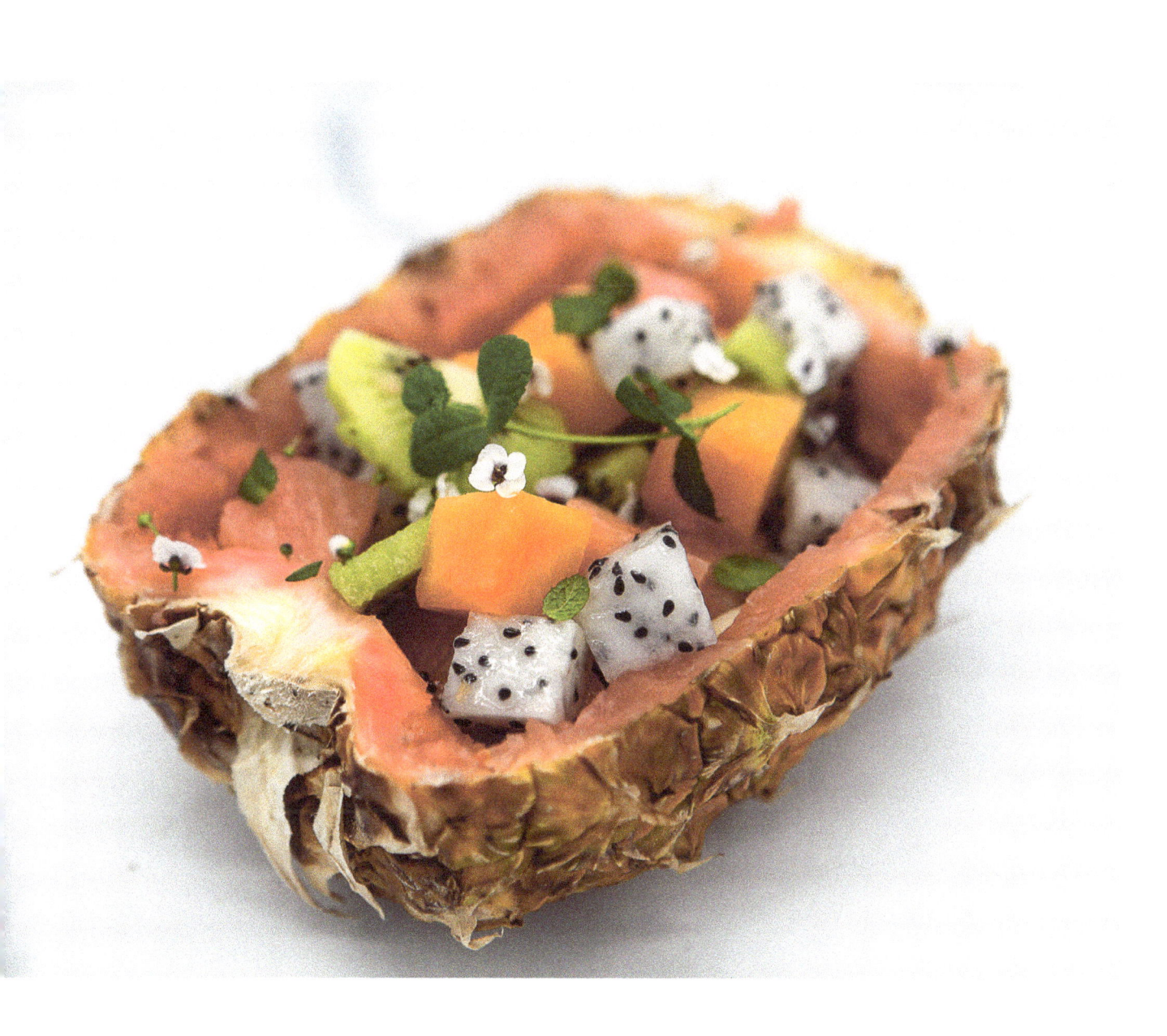

SHRIMP AND MANGO SALAD

PREP TIME 20 minutes, TOTAL TIME 50 minutes
SERVINGS 4 people

INGREDIENTS

- Sea salt and freshly ground black pepper
- 4 black peppercorns
- 2 dried bay leaves
- 1 pound fresh shrimp peeled and deveined
- 1 Mango small, ripe, peeled and diced
- 12 cherry tomatoes, quartered
- 4 tbsp. chopped red onion
- 4 tbsp. olive oil
- 4 tbsp. fresh lime or lemon
- 2 tbsp. fresh orange juice
- 4 tbsp. chopped fresh cilantro or flat leaf parsley
- 2 tbsp. chopped fresh oregano or thyme
- 1/4 tsp. Dijon mustard
- 1 pkg Lettuce Mix
- 1 ripe avocado

INSTRUCTIONS

1. Cook the shrimp: In a pot, combine 1 quart water with 1 tbsp. salt. Add peppercorns and bay leaves and bring to a boil over high heat.

2. Prepare an ice bath: Add enough ice to a large bowl until half full. Sprinkle the ice with 2 tbsp. salt, and top with enough cold water to cover. Set aside.

3. When the water boils, stir the shrimp into the hot water and turn off the heat. Let cook until just pink and opaque for 1-2 minutes, depending on size of shrimp. Drain shrimp and transfer to the ice bath. Stir well and set aside until shrimp are completely chilled, 3 to 5 minutes. Drain shrimp again, and transfer to towels to dry.

4. Make the dressing: In a medium bowl, stir together tomatoes, red onion, oil, fruit juices, herbs, and mustard—season to taste with salt and pepper. Set aside 1/2 of the dressing. In first half of the dressing, add shrimp and mango, toss to coat, and chill for at least 30 minutes (or up to 1 day).

5. When ready to serve, toss the lettuce with the 2nd half of the dressing. Peel and dice the avocado, and toss both into the shrimp salad. Serve chilled in a serving bowl or on individual plates lined with lettuce leaves. Enjoy!

Nurturing Mind, Body, and Soul | *61*

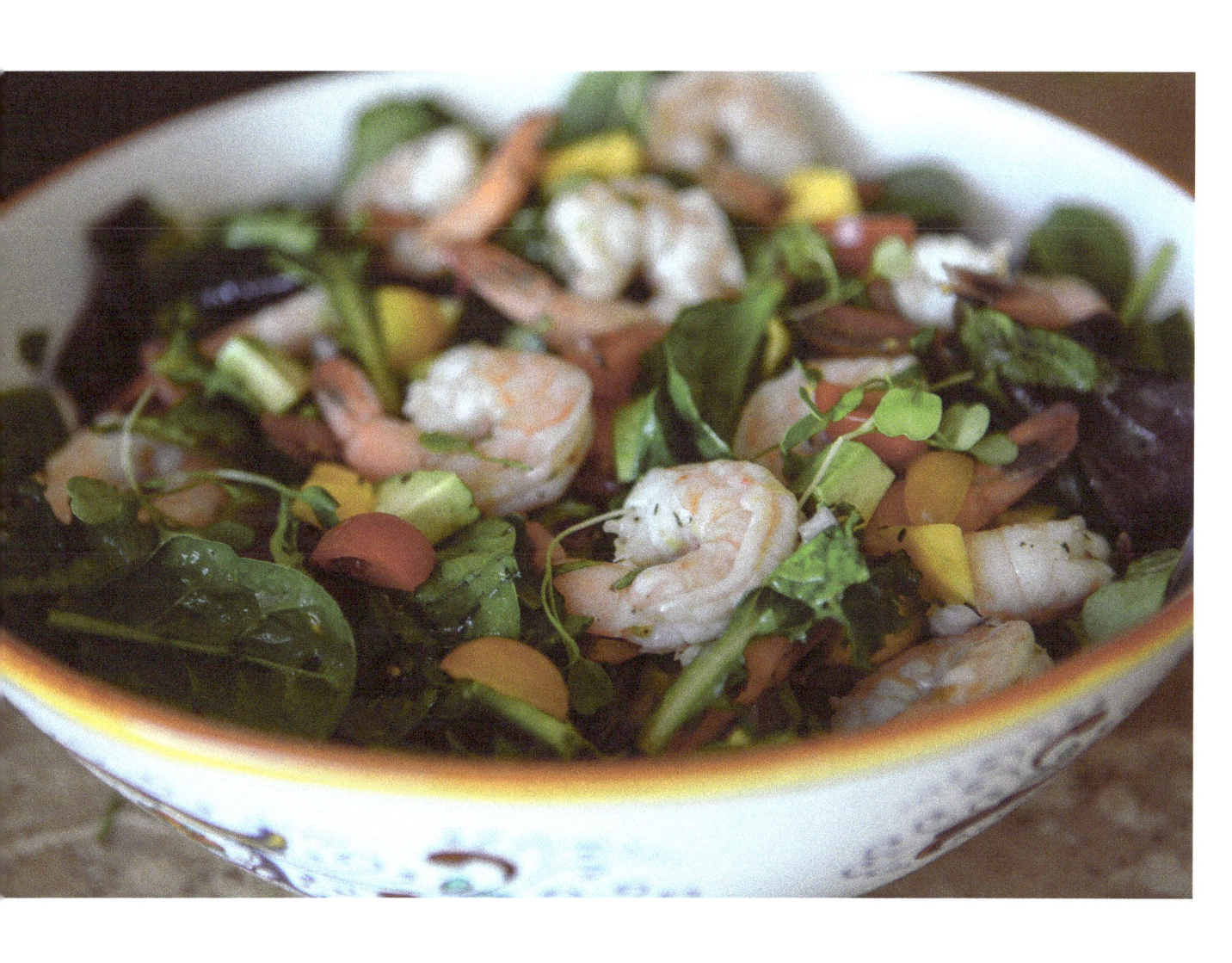

BLOOD ORANGE, FENNEL, AND BURRATA SALAD

Earthy, bittersweet blood oranges have a short season in late winter. I like to take advantage of that time to enjoy their bounty. This blood orange salad takes pungent, delicious ingredients and throws them into a vibrant dish that will delight your taste buds and visual senses. This recipe also works with navel oranges and tangerines, so no worries if you don't have access to blood oranges in your area. This recipe is inspired by Yotam Ottolenghi's in his cookbook *NOPI*. Enjoy!

PREP TIME 8 minutes, COOK TIME 2 minutes
TOTAL TIME 10 minutes, SERVINGS 4 people

INGREDIENTS

- 2 tbsp. extra virgin olive oil
- 1 tsp. Lemon juice
- 1 tsp. honey
- 1 tsp. water
- 1/2 small clove garlic, grated crushed
- 1 bulb fennel sliced paper thin
- 4-5 blood oranges/naval oranges a combination
- 1-2 burrata balls (or 4 separate ones if you're making separate plates per person)
- Coarse sea salt
- Ground black pepper

To Dressing

- 1-2 tbsp. pistachios chopped
- 1-2 tbsp. micro greens
- Fennel fronds optional

INSTRUCTIONS

Dressing

1. Heat the oil on medium-low in a small saucepan with honey, water, garlic, and a tsp. of salt.
2. Remove once it begins to simmer.
3. Stir in lemon juice, remove the garlic clove and set aside.

Salad

1. Cut the fronds off the fennel and slice the rest thinly with a mandolin or vegetable peeler.
2. Add the fennel to a bowl, dress with a squeeze of fresh orange juice, and season with salt and pepper.
3. On a platter (or four separate smaller plates), spread a layer of the fennel.
4. Trim off the tops and bottoms from the oranges.
5. Cut down the sides of the oranges, following their natural curve, to remove the skin and white pith. Cut into 1/2 to 3/4 inch slices.

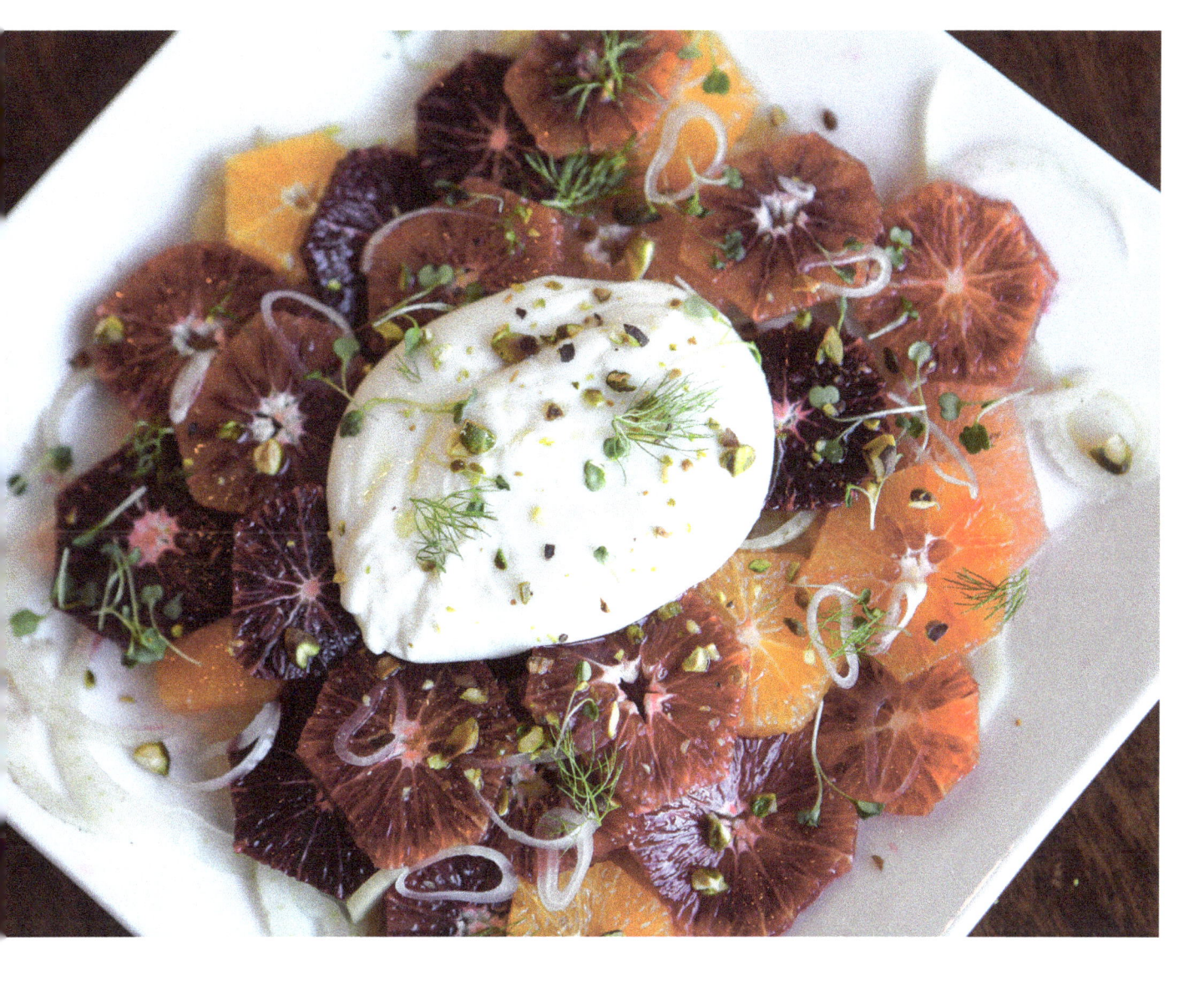

6. Divide the orange slices over the plate(s), slightly overlapping, on top of the fennel, and place a burrata ball on top.

7. Spoon the dressing over the cheese and oranges.

8. Top with chopped pistachios, micro-greens, fennel fronds, and a few thin slices of fennel to serve. Enjoy!

MICROGREENS SALAD

Prep TIME 15 minutes, TOTAL TIME 15 minutes
SERVINGS 4 people

INGREDIENTS

- 2 cups mixed microgreens such as arugula, kale, beet greens, or radish greens
- 1 cup fresh strawberries diced
- 1 cup cucumber diced
- 1/4 cup crumbled feta cheese optional
- 1/4 cup chopped pecans optional

For the Dressing:

- 3 tbsp. extra-virgin olive oil
- 1 tbsp. balsamic vinegar
- 1 tbsp. orange juice
- 1 tsp. dijon mustard optional
- 1 clove garlic optional
- Salt and pepper to taste

INSTRUCTIONS

1. Wash the microgreens thoroughly and pat them dry using a clean kitchen towel or paper towel. Place the micro-greens in a large salad bowl.

2. Wash the strawberries and cucumber. Remove the stems from the strawberries and dice them. Dice the cucumber, depending on your preference. Add the diced strawberries and cucumber to the salad bowl with the microgreens.

3. Crumble the feta cheese over the salad. If you prefer goat cheese, you can also crumble that over the salad.

4. If using, chop the pecans and sprinkle them over the salad for extra texture and flavor.

5. In a separate small bowl, whisk together the extra-virgin olive oil, balsamic vinegar, honey, and Dijon mustard (if using) to make the dressing. Season the dressing with salt and pepper to taste.

6. Pour the dressing over the salad and gently toss everything together until the ingredients are well combined and coated.

7. Serve the salad immediately as a refreshing appetizer or a light main course. It's perfect for a summer lunch or dinner! Enjoy!

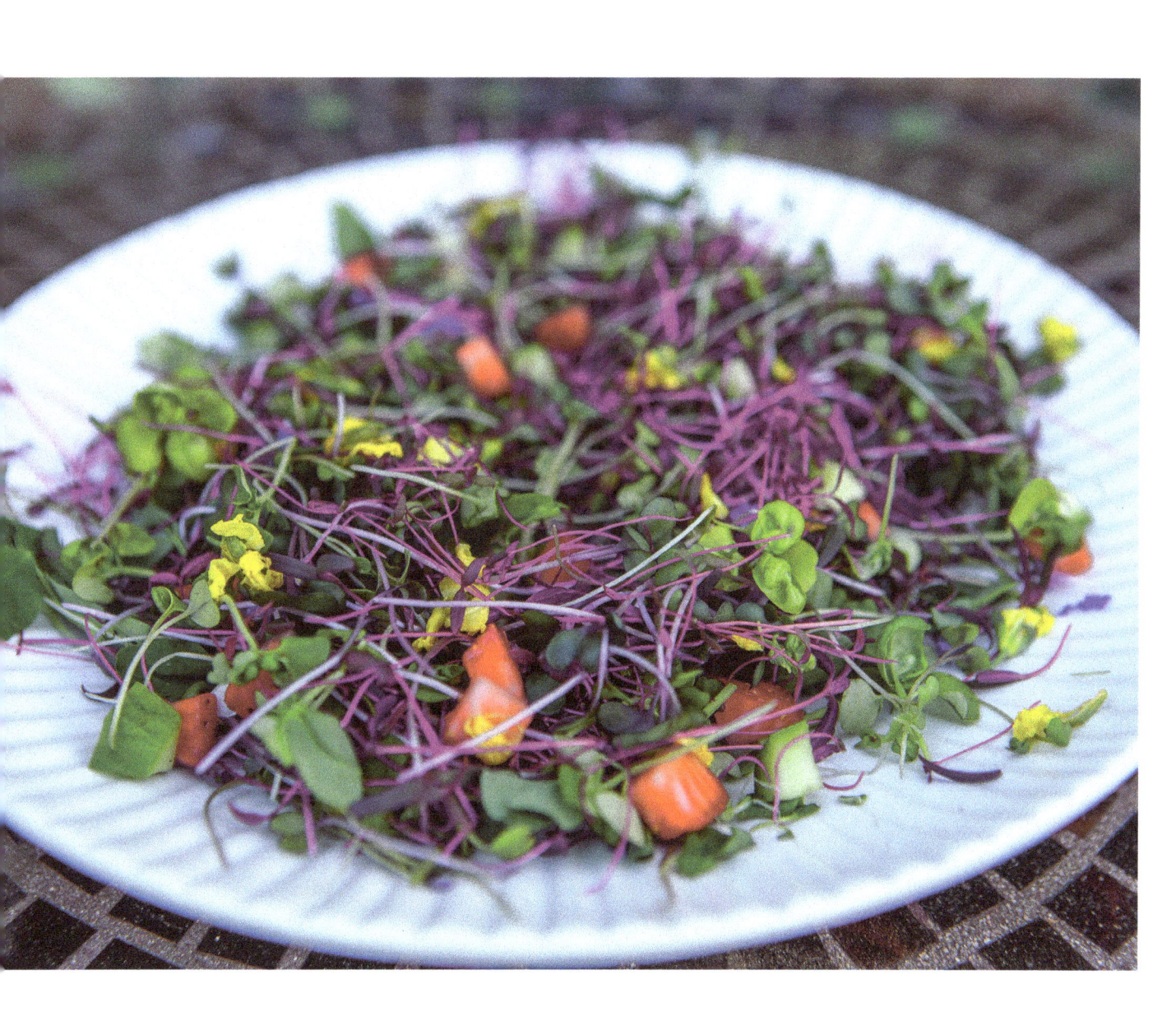

LEMON AND CHICKPEA SOUP

This soup is vibrant, with the tanginess of lemon and the earthiness of chickpeas and spices. It's a comforting yet refreshing dish, perfect for any season!

PREP TIME 10 minutes, COOK TIME 20 minutes, TOTAL TIME 30 minutes, SERVINGS 4 people

INGREDIENTS

- 2 tbsp. olive oil
- 1 medium onion finely chopped
- Garlic minced: 3 cloves
- 2 medium carrots sliced
- 2 celery stalks diced
- 1 tsp. ground cumin
- 1 tsp. ground coriander
- 1/2 tsp. turmeric
- 2 cups chickpeas cooked or canned drained and rinsed
- 4 cups vegetable or chicken broth
- 2 Lemons juice of
- Salt and pepper to taste
- Fresh parsley or cilantro chopped for garnish
- Lemon slices for garnish

INSTRUCTIONS

1. In a large pot, heat the olive oil over medium heat. Add the chopped onion, garlic, carrots, and celery. Sauté until the vegetables are tender, about 5 minutes.
2. Stir in the ground cumin, coriander, and turmeric. Cook for another minute until the spices are fragrant.
3. Add the chickpeas to the pot. Pour in the vegetable broth and bring the mixture to a boil. Reduce heat and simmer for about 15 minutes.
4. For a creamier texture, take out about a cup of the soup and blend it until smooth, then return it to the pot. This step is optional.
5. Stir in the fresh lemon juice—season with salt and pepper to taste.
6. Ladle the soup into bowls. Garnish with fresh parsley or cilantro and a slice of lemon.
7. Serve hot, ideally with a slice of crusty bread or a side salad for a complete meal.

Nutrition for the Mind, Body, and Soul | 67

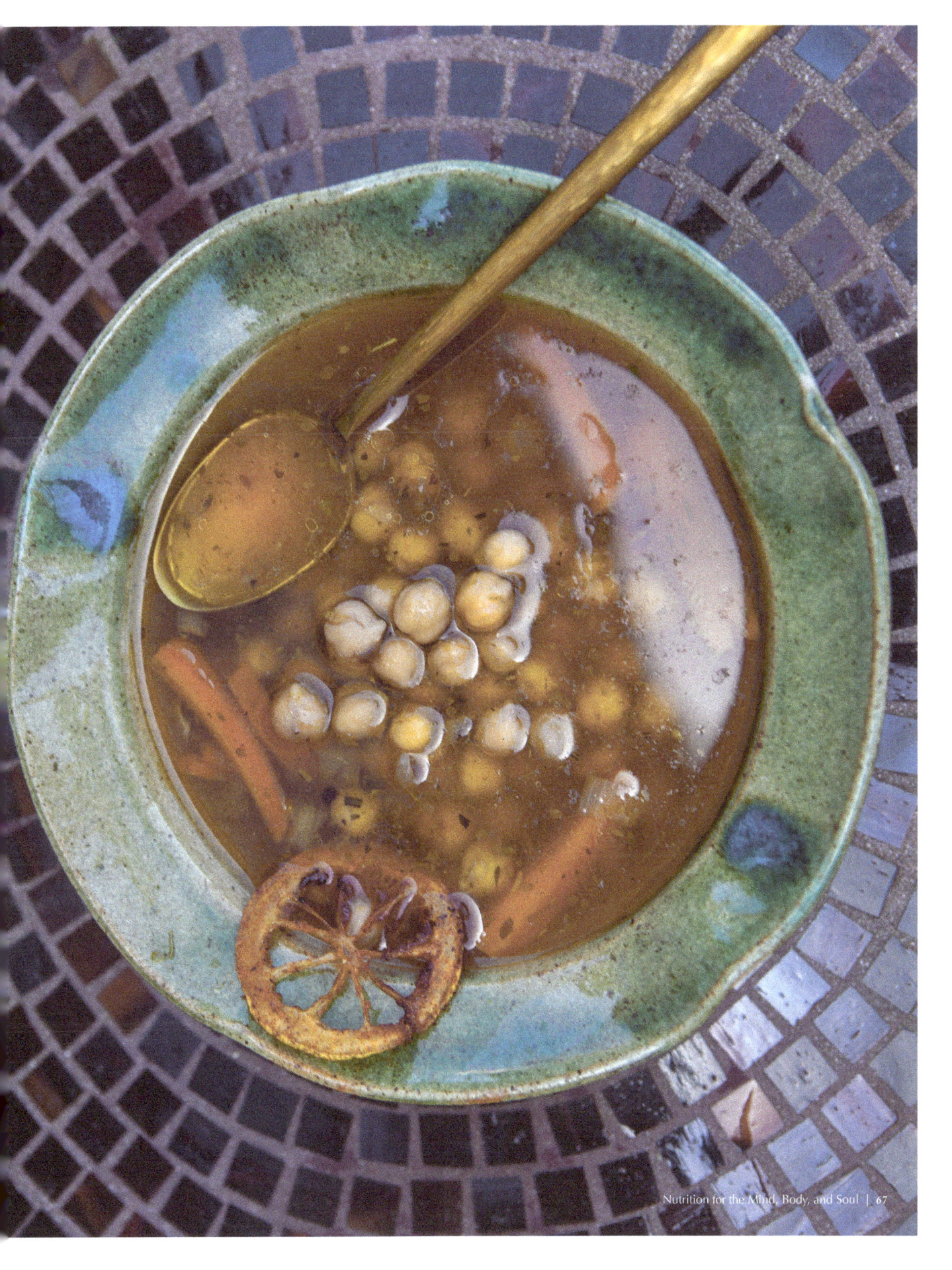

BUTTERNUT SQUASH SOUP WITH WILD MUSHROOMS AND MISO

This luxurious Butternut Squash Soup is a harmonious blend of earthy, sweet, and savory notes that will transport your taste buds to a place of comforting indulgence.

PREP TIME 25 minutes, COOK TIME 25 minutes, TOTAL TIME 50 minutes, SERVINGS 6 bowls

INGREDIENTS

For the Soup

- 2 lbs. about 1 kg. of butternut squash, peeled, seeded, and diced
- 1 onion chopped
- 2 cloves garlic minced
- 1 tbsp. olive oil
- 4 cups vegetable broth
- 1/4 cup white miso paste
- 1/2 cup plain greek yogurt optional for creaminess
- Salt and black pepper to taste

For the Wild Mushrooms

- 8 oz. about 225 grams of mixed wild mushrooms (such as shiitake, oyster, or cremini), cleaned and sliced
- 2 tbsp. olive oil
- 2 cloves garlic minced
- Salt and black pepper to taste
- Fresh thyme leaves for garnish

INSTRUCTIONS

For the Soup

1. In a large soup pot, heat 1 tbsp. of olive oil over medium heat. Add the chopped onion and sauté for about 5 minutes or until translucent.

2. Add the minced garlic and sauté for another 1-2 minutes until fragrant.

3. Add the diced squash to the pot and sauté for 5 minutes, stirring occasionally.

4. Pour in the vegetable broth and bring the mixture to a boil. Reduce the heat to low, cover, and simmer for 20-25 minutes or until the pumpkin/squash is tender and easily pierced with a fork.

5. Mix the white miso paste with a few tbsp. of the soup broth in a small bowl to create a smooth paste.

6. Remove the soup pot from the heat and let it cool slightly. Then, using an immersion blender or countertop blender, puree the soup until smooth.

NOTES

Serve your Butternut Squash Soup hot and enjoy the rich, comforting flavors!

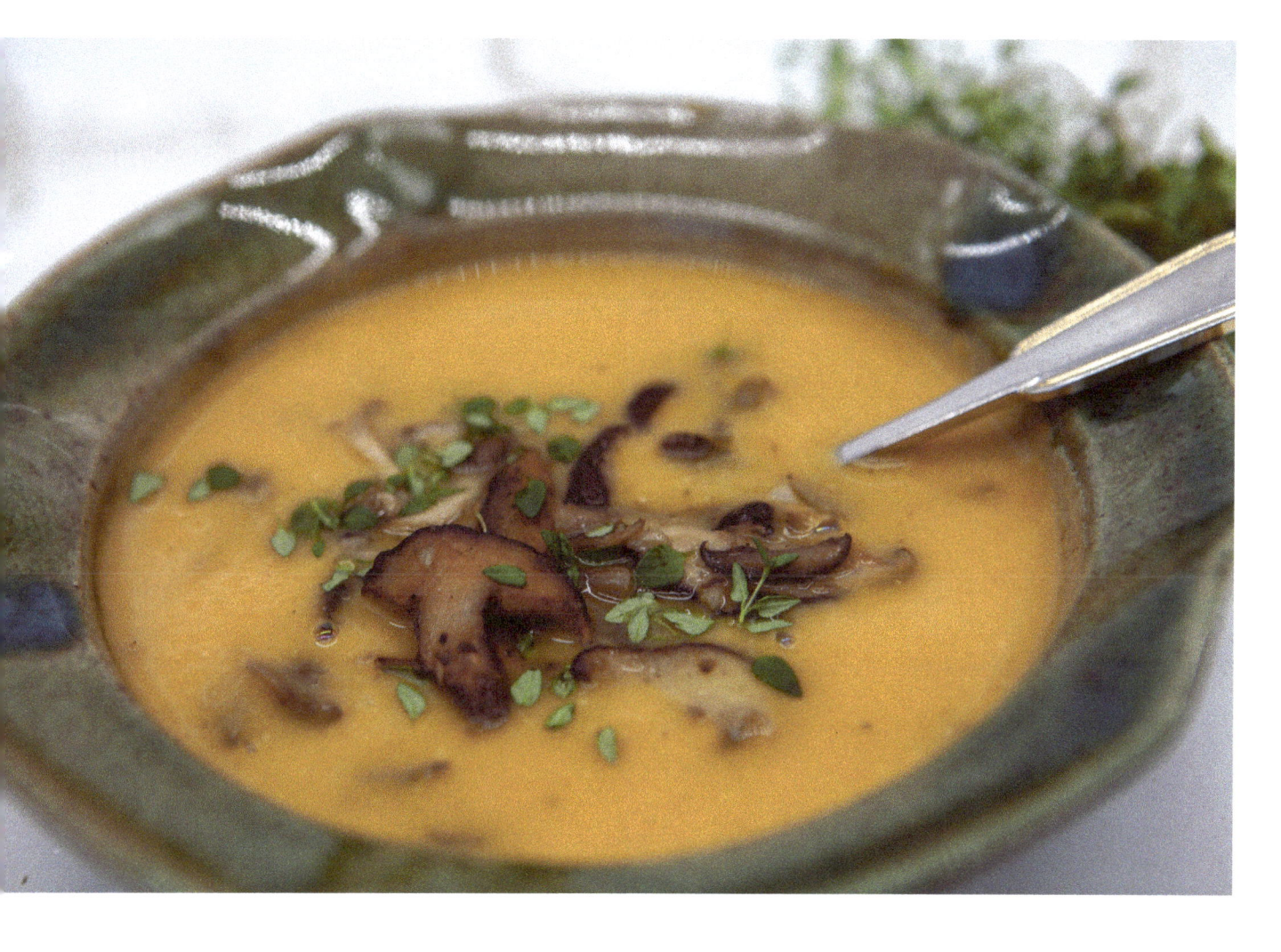

7. Return the pureed soup to the pot and stir in the miso paste mixture and Greek yogurt (if using)—season with salt and black pepper to taste. Simmer for an additional 5 minutes to heat through.

For the Wild Mushrooms

1. While the soup is simmering, heat 2 tbsp. of olive oil in a separate skillet over medium-high heat.
2. Add the minced garlic and sliced wild mushrooms to the skillet. Sauté for about 5-7 minutes, or until the mushrooms are tender and browned.
3. Season the mushrooms with salt and black pepper to taste, and remove them from the heat.

To Serve

Ladle the hot pumpkin (or squash) soup into bowls. Top each serving with a generous portion of sautéed wild mushrooms and a sprinkle of fresh thyme leaves for garnish.

PEAR AND GOAT CHEESE APPETIZER

Baked Pear and Goat Cheese Appetizer with Pine Nuts, and Olive Oil Honey Dressing. This dish combines sweet, savory, and herbal flavors for a truly delightful appetizer. The herbed olive oil with garlic and honey adds a wonderful aromatic quality to the sweet pears, while the goat cheese and pine nuts provide creamy and nutty notes. Finished with a drizzle of honey, which brings out the subtle sweet notes.

*PREP TIME 20 minutes, COOK TIME 45-55 minutes,
TOTAL TIME 75 minutes, SERVINGS 8 pear halves*

INGREDIENTS

- 4 ripe but firm pears (like bosc or anjou)
- 100 g. soft goat cheese
- 1/4 cup pine nuts

For the Herbed Olive Oil Dressing

- 1/2 cup olive oil
- 2 cloves garlic, minced
- 1 tbsp. honey
- 1 tbsp. fresh herbs (like thyme, rosemary, or parsley), finely chopped
- Salt and pepper to taste

INSTRUCTIONS

1. Preheat your oven to 375°F.
2. Prepare the Dressing. In a small bowl, whisk together olive oil, minced garlic, honey, chopped herbs, salt, and pepper. Set aside.
3. Prepare Pears. Cut the pears in half and use a melon baller to remove the cores.
4. Place the pear halves on a baking sheet.
5. Brush the herbed olive oil dressing generously over the cut sides of the pears.
6. Fill the holes of each pear half with goat cheese. Sprinkle with pine nuts.
7. Place in the oven and bake for about 45-55 minutes, or until the pears are tender and lightly browned.
8. Serve. Let the pears cool for a few minutes. Drizzle honey with honey and sprinkle with fresh thyme. Serve warm as an appetizer. Enjoy!

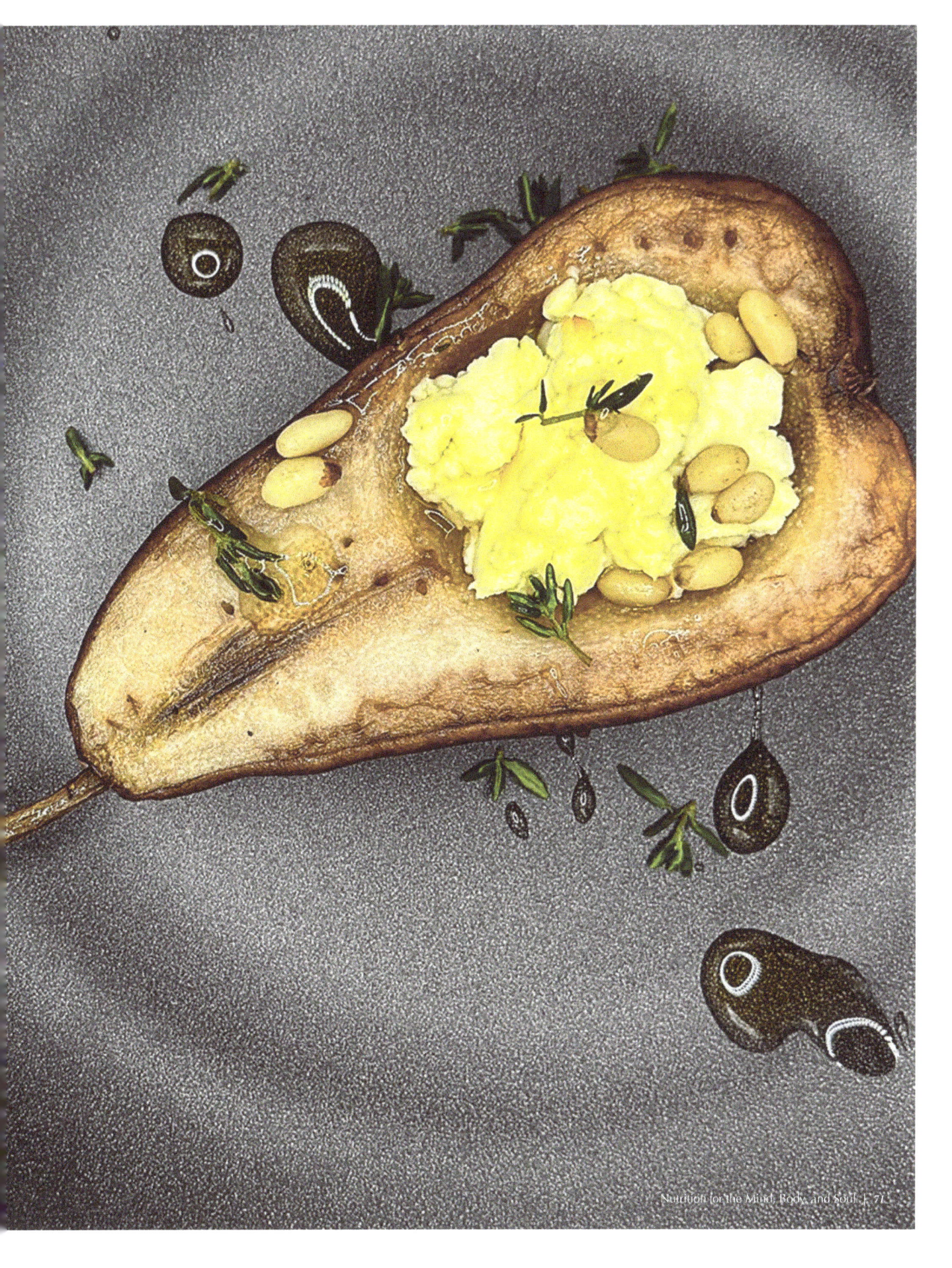

TOMATO TART

PREP TIME 10 minutes, COOK TIME 25 minutes
TOTAL TIME 35 minutes, SERVINGS 6 tarts

INGREDIENTS

- all-purpose flour for dusting gluten free flour is okay here.
- 1 sheet puff pastry gluten free or regular—thawed.
- 2 tbsp. parmesan cheese
- kosher salt & freshly ground black peppercorns to taste
- 1 large egg
- 15 assorted heirloom cherry or grape tomatoes sliced halfwise
- 2 tbsp. extra virgin olive oil plus additional for drizzle
- fresh basil or thyme leaves thinly sliced for garnish

INSTRUCTIONS

1. Heat oven to 350 degrees. Lightly dust work surface and puff pastry with flour. Roll pastry to 15-inches by 10-inches and cut into six 5-inch circles. Place on a parchment lined baking sheet and set aside.

2. In a small bowl whisk egg. Split egg into two separate bowls and add the Parmesan cheese, salt and pepper to one of the bowls and stir to combine. Set aside remaining egg portion.

3. Evenly divide the egg and parmesan cheese mixture among the six pastry squares and spread to within 1-inch of the edges. Brush the edges with reserved egg. Evenly divide tomatoes and drizzle with olive oil.

4. Bake 25-30 minutes, rotating pan halfway through, until pastry is puffed and golden. Garnish with basil or thyme and drizzle with additional olive oil.

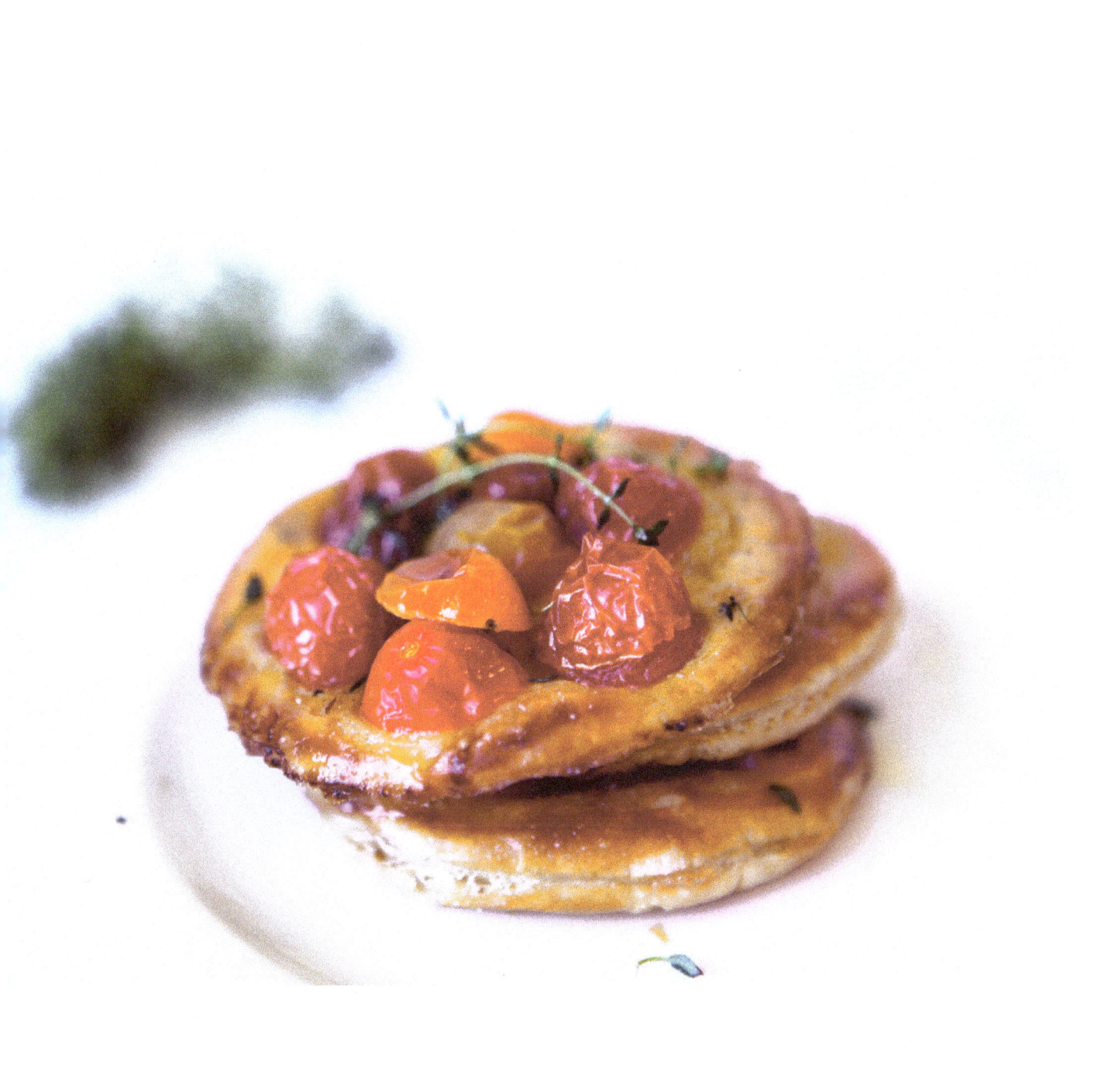

WILD MUSHROOMS AND CREAMY POLENTA

This dish is a comforting earthy delight that brings out the deep flavors of wild mushrooms.

PREP TIME 20 minutes, COOK TIME 30 minutes, TOTAL TIME 50 minutes, SERVINGS 4 people

INGREDIENTS

For the Mushrooms

- 1 lbs. wild mushrooms like chanterelles, porcini, morels, etc., cleaned and sliced
- 2 cloves garlic finely minced
- 2 tbsp. unsalted butter vegan: sub with olive oil or high-quality vegan butter or margarine.
- 2 tbsp. olive oil
- 1/4 cup white wine optional
- 2 tbsp. fresh thyme leaves
- Salt and pepper to taste
- Fresh parsley finely chopped (for garnish)
- Grated parmesan or pecorino cheese optional for garnish. vegan: sub with a vegan parmesan alternative, found in health food stores, or nutritional yeast for a cheesy flavor.

For the Polenta

- 1 cup polenta or grits
- 4 cups chicken or vegetable broth you can also use water, but broth gives more flavor
- 1/2 cup grated parmesan cheese vegan: sub with a vegan parmesan alternative, found in health food stores, or nutritional yeast for a cheesy flavor.
- 2 tbsp. unsalted butter vegan: sub with high-quality vegan butter or margarine
- Salt to taste

INSTRUCTIONS

Prepare the Creamy Polenta

1. In a medium saucepan, bring the broth to a boil.
2. Gradually whisk in the polenta or grits. Reduce heat to low and simmer, stirring often, until the mixture thickens and the polenta is tender. This will take about 20-25 minutes for polenta and about 5-10 minutes for grits.
3. Stir in the butter, parmesan cheese. Season with salt. If the mixture becomes too thick, you can add a bit more broth or water to reach your desired consistency. Keep warm.

Cook the Wild Mushrooms

1. In a large skillet over medium heat, melt butter with olive oil. Once heated, add the sliced wild mushrooms.
2. Cook, stirring occasionally, until the mushrooms release their moisture and start to brown, about 8-10 minutes.

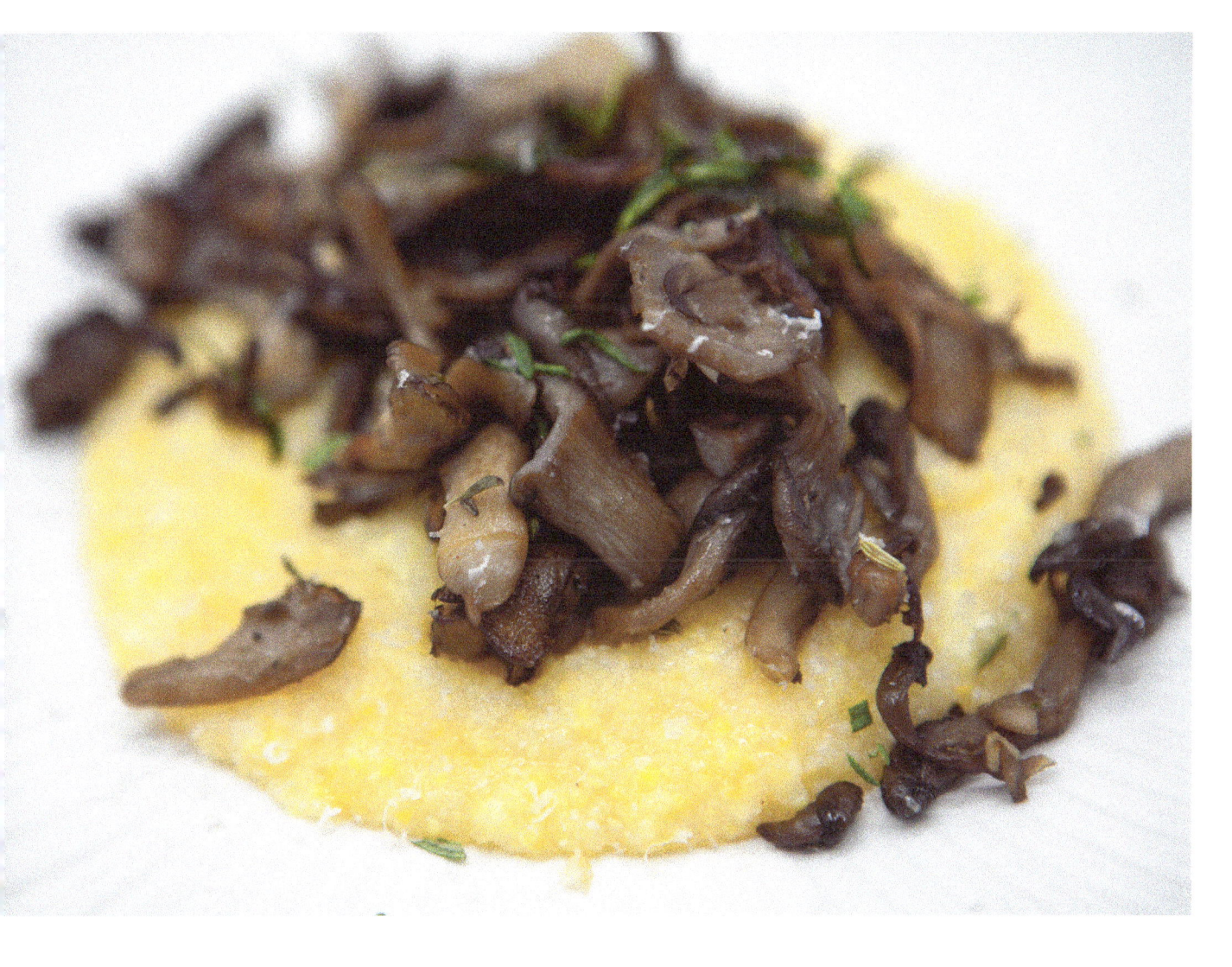

3. Add the minced garlic and fresh thyme leaves. Continue to cook for another 2 minutes until the garlic is fragrant.

4. If using wine, pour it into the skillet to deglaze, scraping up any brown bits from the bottom. Allow the wine to reduce by half.

5. Season with salt and pepper.

Assemble and Serve

1. Spoon the creamy polenta or grits onto plates or a serving dish.

2. Top with the sautéed wild mushrooms.

3. Garnish with fresh parsley and optionally, more grated cheese.

4. Serve hot and enjoy the delicious harmony of earthy wild mushrooms and the creamy texture of the polenta or grits.

SPRING HERB FRITTATA

This herb frittata will brighten up any Spring table. Enjoy the freshness of this nutritious dish with family and loved ones.

PREP TIME 20 minutes, COOK TIME 20 minutes, RESTING TIME 5 minutes
TOTAL TIME 45 minutes, SERVINGS 6 people

INGREDIENTS

- 1/4 cup sour cream you can substitue crème fraîche or plain greek yogurt.
- 2 tbsp. chopped chives
- 6 large eggs
- 6 scallions cut into 1-in. pieces
- 2 cup flat-leaf parsley leaves plus more for sprinkling
- 2 cups cilantro and more for sprinkling
- 1/2 cup dill fronds plus more for sprinkling
- 2 tbsp. tarragon leaves plus more for sprinkling
- 4 tbsp. olive oil divided
- Salt and pepper

INSTRUCTIONS

1. Heat oven to 350°F. In a small bowl, stir together crème fraîche and chives; set aside.
2. In large bowl, lightly beat eggs. In a food processor, pulse scallions, parsley, cilantro, dill, tarragon and 2 tbsp. oil until evenly and finely chopped. Add to bowl with eggs along with 1/2 tsp. each salt and pepper and mix to combine.
3. Heat remaining 2 tbsp. oil in medium skillet on medium until shimmering, about 2 minutes.
4. Add egg mixture and cook until edges have begun to sizzle and set, about 2 minutes.
5. Transfer the skillet to the oven and bake until the center is just set, 18 to 20 minutes.
6. Let rest at least 5 minutes.
7. Serve with chive crème fraîche or sour cream. Sprinkle with more herbs, if desired.

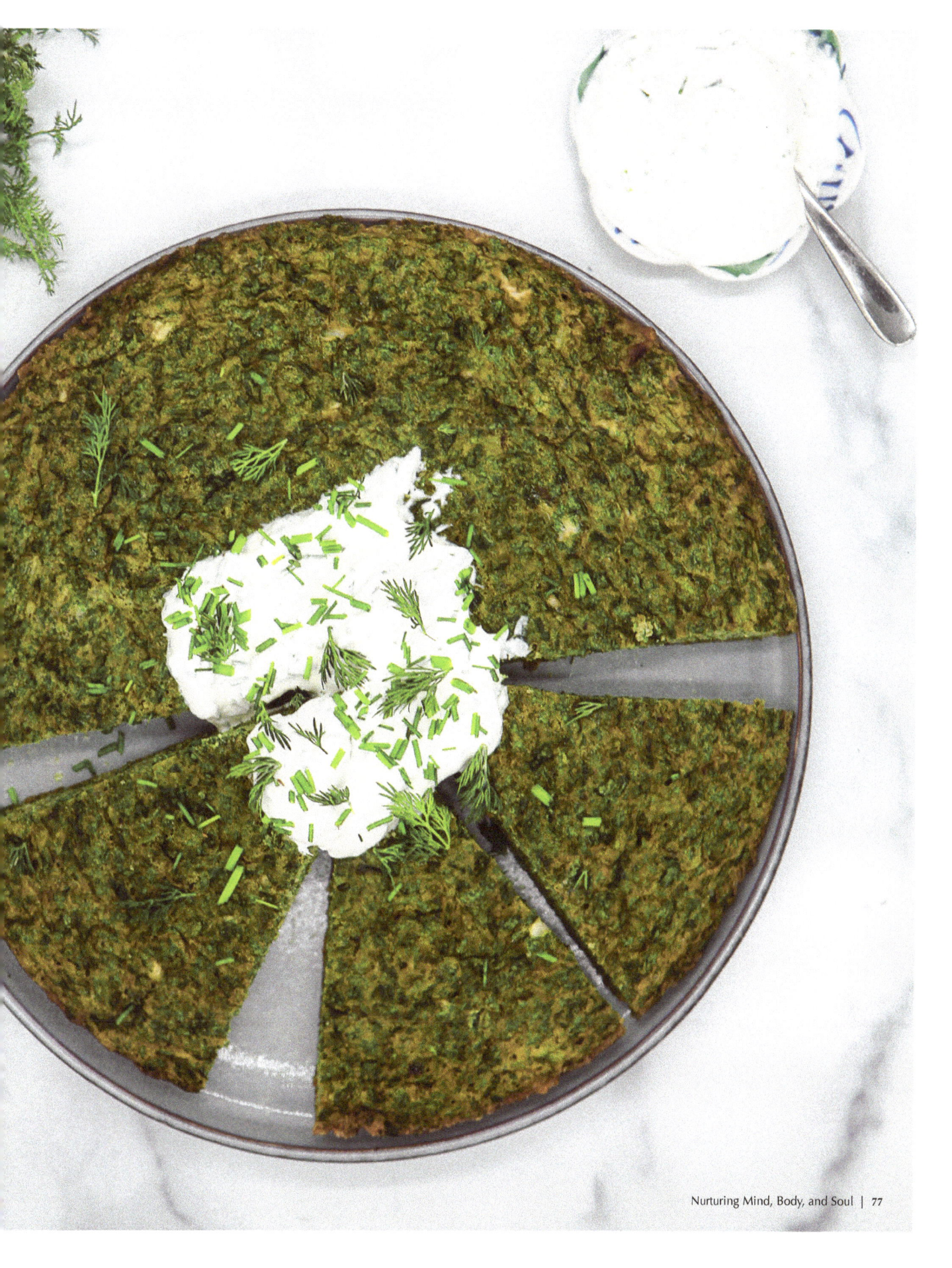

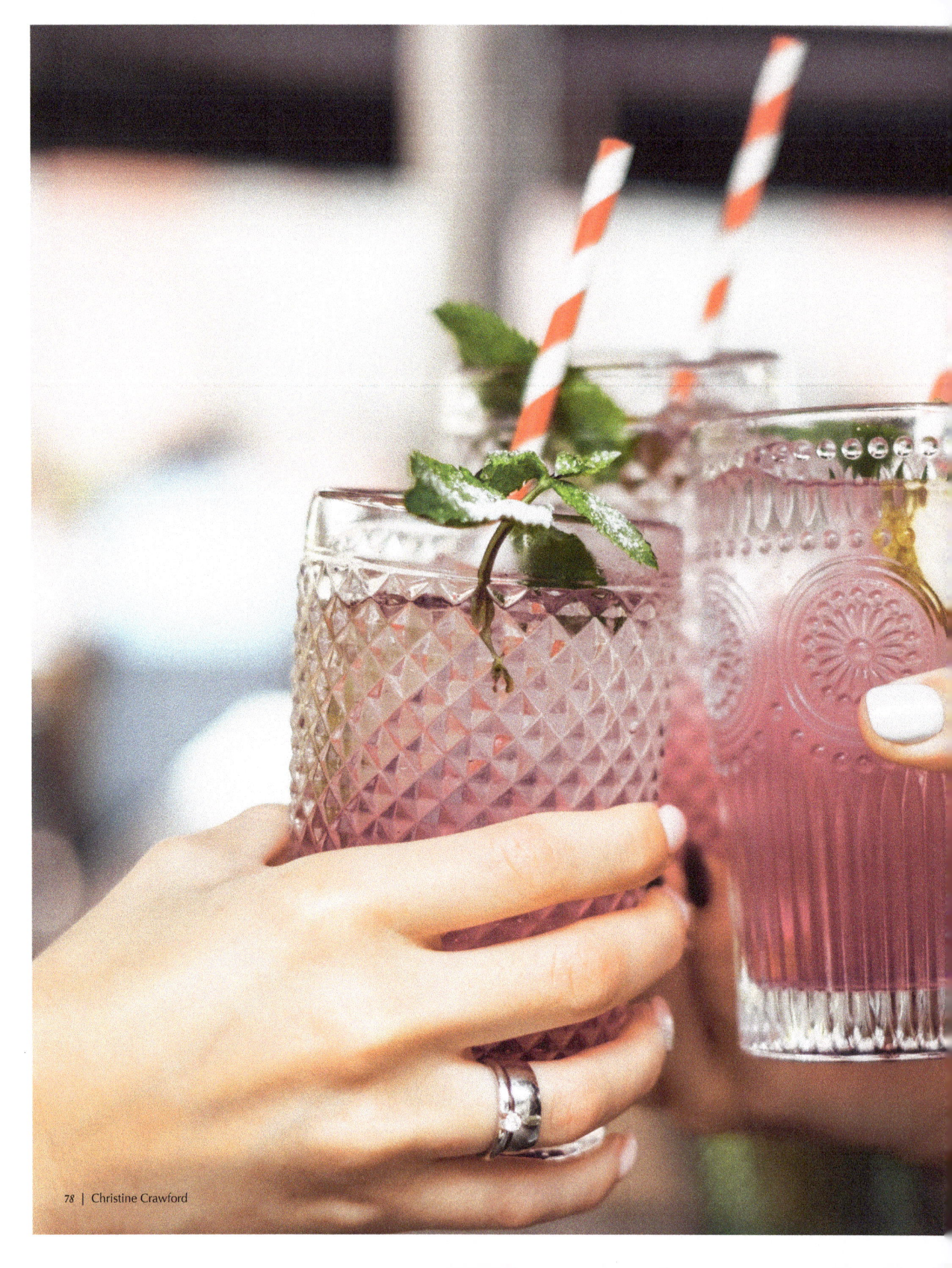

MOCKTAILS

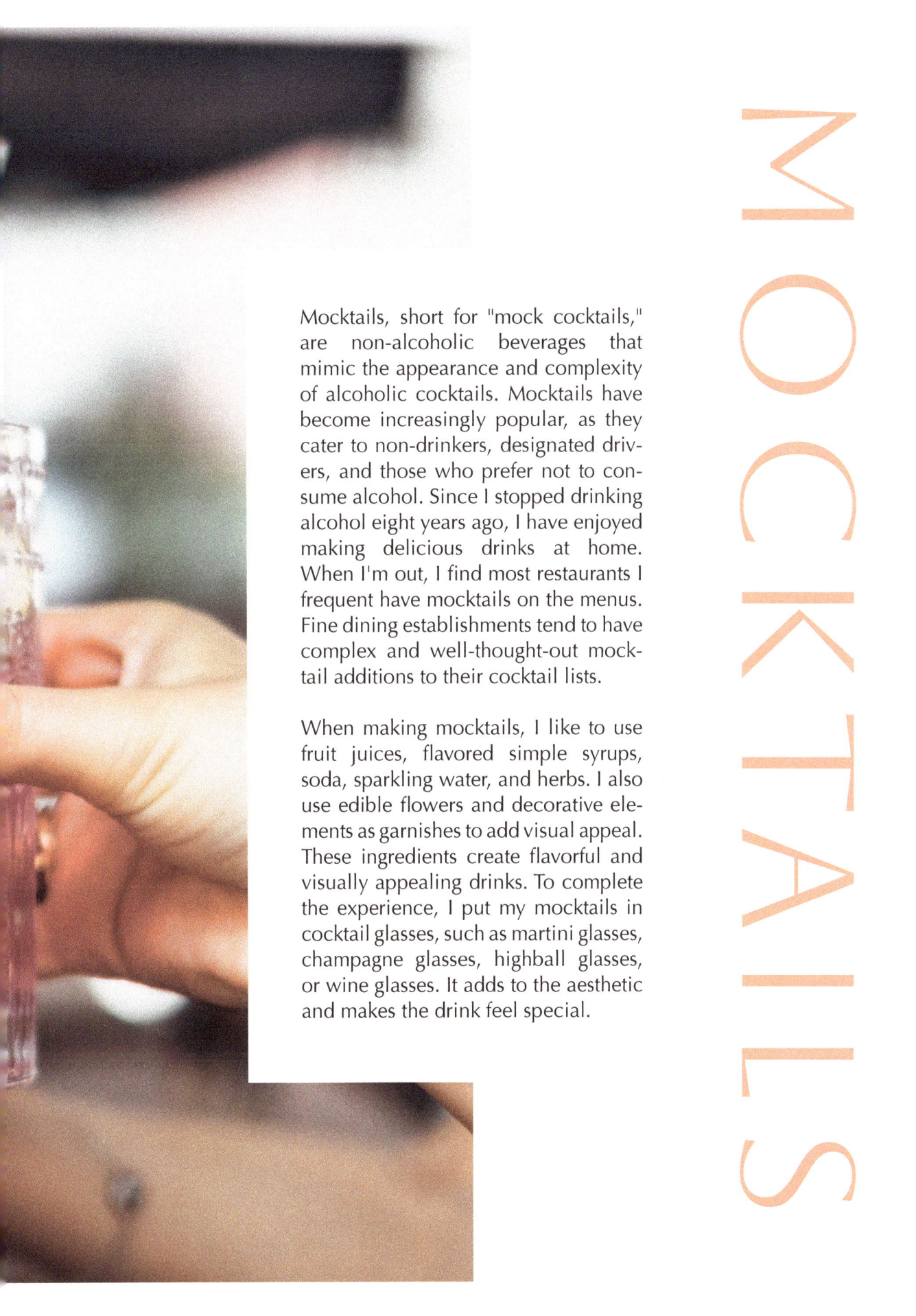

Mocktails, short for "mock cocktails," are non-alcoholic beverages that mimic the appearance and complexity of alcoholic cocktails. Mocktails have become increasingly popular, as they cater to non-drinkers, designated drivers, and those who prefer not to consume alcohol. Since I stopped drinking alcohol eight years ago, I have enjoyed making delicious drinks at home. When I'm out, I find most restaurants I frequent have mocktails on the menus. Fine dining establishments tend to have complex and well-thought-out mocktail additions to their cocktail lists.

When making mocktails, I like to use fruit juices, flavored simple syrups, soda, sparkling water, and herbs. I also use edible flowers and decorative elements as garnishes to add visual appeal. These ingredients create flavorful and visually appealing drinks. To complete the experience, I put my mocktails in cocktail glasses, such as martini glasses, champagne glasses, highball glasses, or wine glasses. It adds to the aesthetic and makes the drink feel special.

ROSE LEMON SPARKLER

PREP TIME 5 minutes, COOK TIME 5 minutes
CHILLING TIME 30 minutes, TOTAL TIME 40 minutes
SERVINGS 8 drinks

EQUIPMENT

- Juicer
- Sauce pan
- Pitcher

INGREDIENTS

- 1 cup rosewater
- 1 hibiscus tea bag
- 1/4 cup maple syrup
- 3 lemons
- 6 cups sparkling water

INSTRUCTIONS

1. Make Rose Hibiscus Simple Syrup:
2. Combine the rose water, maple syrup, and hibiscus tea bag in a saucepan.
3. Bring to a boil, then immediately turn off the heat.
4. Let it sit for 5 minutes.
5. Cool to room temperature.
6. Squeeze the tea bag and remove it.
7. Refrigerate.
8. After the syrup is chilled, add the lemon juice to a pitcher and stir in the rose syrup.
9. Top up with sparkling water and stir well. Taste, and add more rose syrup or lemon juice if you'd like.

Nurturing Mind, Body, and Soul | 81

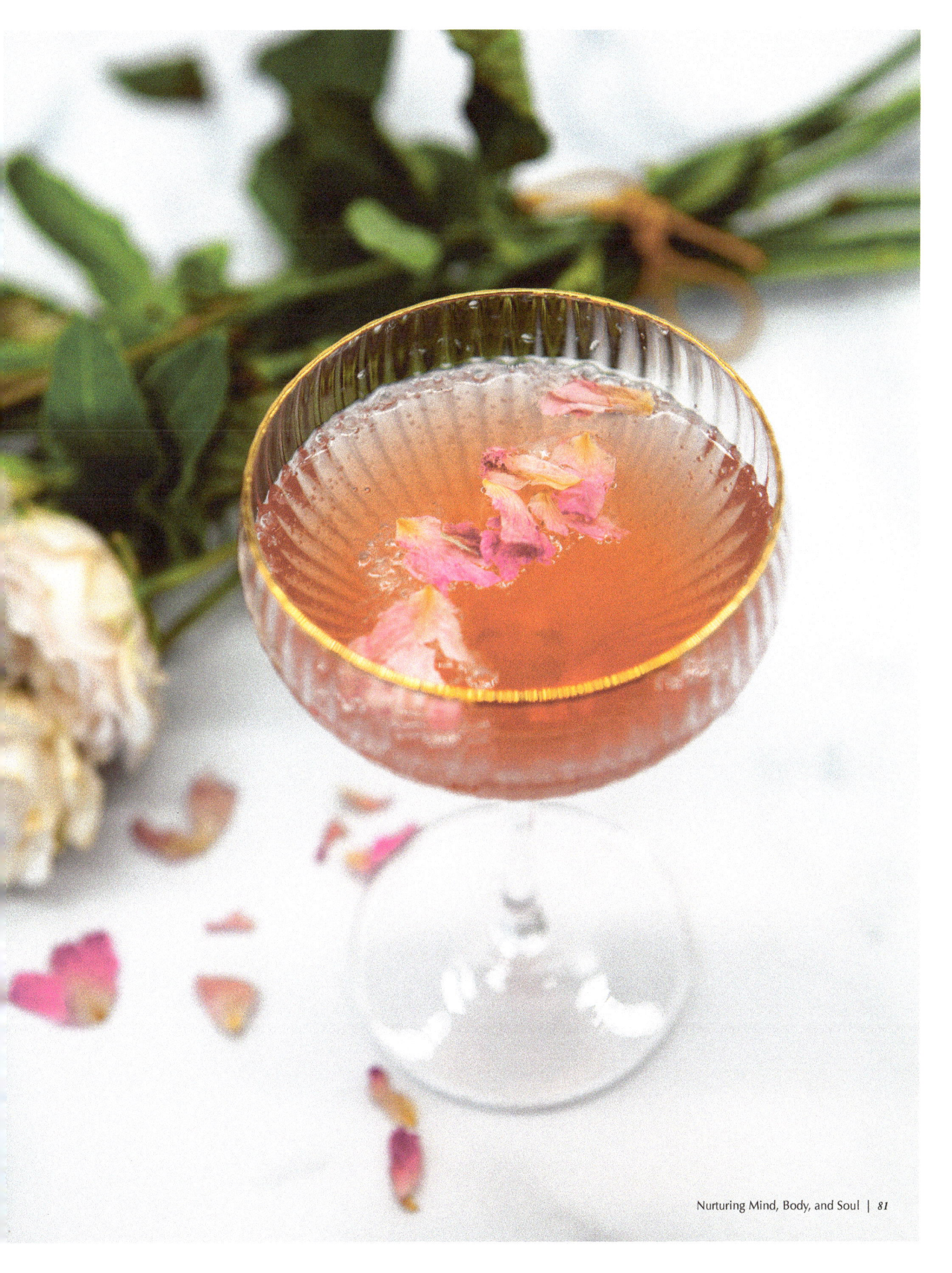

STRAWBERRY LEMONADE

PREP TIME 10 minutes, TOTAL TIME 10 minutes, SERVINGS 4 people

INGREDIENTS

- 3 cups filtered or spring water
- 1 cup diced strawberries
- 1/4 cup medjool dates
- 2 lemons: juice of
- 2-3 sprigs of fresh mint

INSTRUCTIONS

1. Combine all the ingredients (excluding the mint) in a blender.
2. Process until smooth and creamy, roughly 1-2 minutes.
3. Strain the mixture using a fine mesh sieve to filter out any large pieces. While this step is optional, it's advised for a silkier lemonade.
4. Transfer the mixture to a sealed container and including the mint sprigs. Close tightly and refrigerate for about an hour or until it's cold.
5. Serve over ice.

NOTES

For a sweeter lemonade, increase the number of dates. Enjoy!

Nutrition for the Mind, Body, and Soul | 83

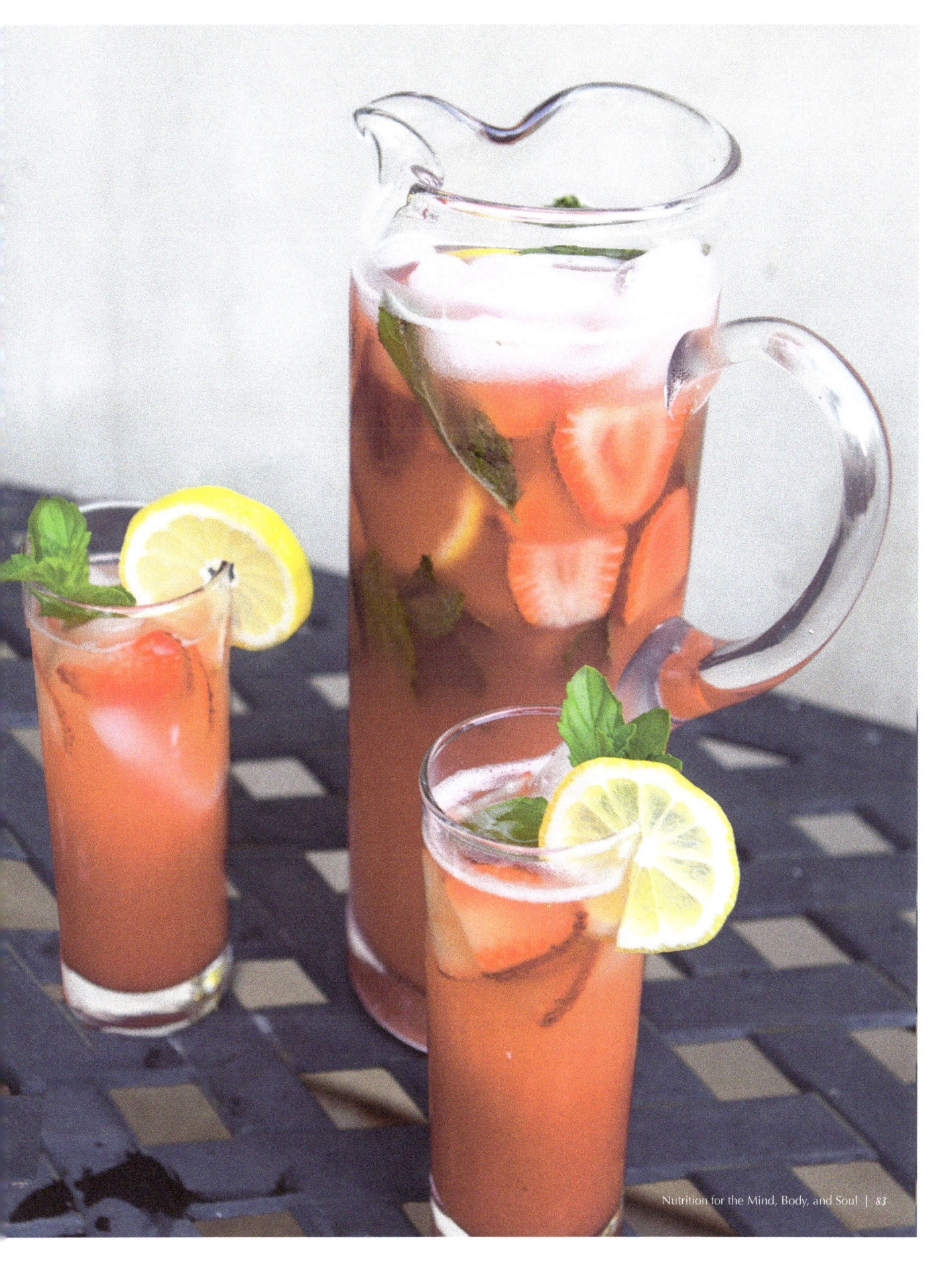

EARL GREY CITRUS MOCKTAIL

This refreshing drink combines the distinct flavor of Earl Grey tea with the citrusy notes of orange and lemon, creating a perfect non-alcoholic beverage for any occasion.

PREP TIME 10 minutes, TOTAL TIME 10 minutes, SERVINGS 4 people

INGREDIENTS

- 3 Earl Grey tea bags
- 1 cup boiling water
- 1/2 cup fresh orange juice
- 1/4 cup fresh lemon juice
- Ice cubes
- Sparkling water or club soda
- Orange and lemon slices for garnish

INSTRUCTIONS

1. Place the Earl Grey tea bags in a heatproof container. Pour 1 cup of boiling water over the tea bags and let them steep for about 5 minutes. After steeping, remove the tea bags and allow the tea to cool to room temperature.
2. In a pitcher, combine the freshly squeezed orange and lemon juices. Add honey or simple syrup to sweeten the mix. Stir well until the honey or syrup is completely dissolved.
3. Once the tea has cooled, add it to the citrus mixture in the pitcher. Stir well to combine.
4. Fill glasses with ice cubes. Pour the tea and citrus mixture over the ice, filling each glass about two-thirds full.
5. Top up each glass with sparkling water or club soda for a refreshing fizz.
6. Add a slice of orange and lemon to each glass. If desired.
7. Stir gently before serving. Enjoy your Earl Grey Citrus Mocktail!
8. This mocktail is perfect for those who love the aromatic flavor of Earl Grey tea, complemented by the zesty freshness of citrus fruits. It's a sophisticated and enjoyable drink for any time of the day!

NOTES

If you prefer your drink sweeter you can add 2 tbsp. of maple syrup.

Nurturing Mind, Body, and Soul | 85

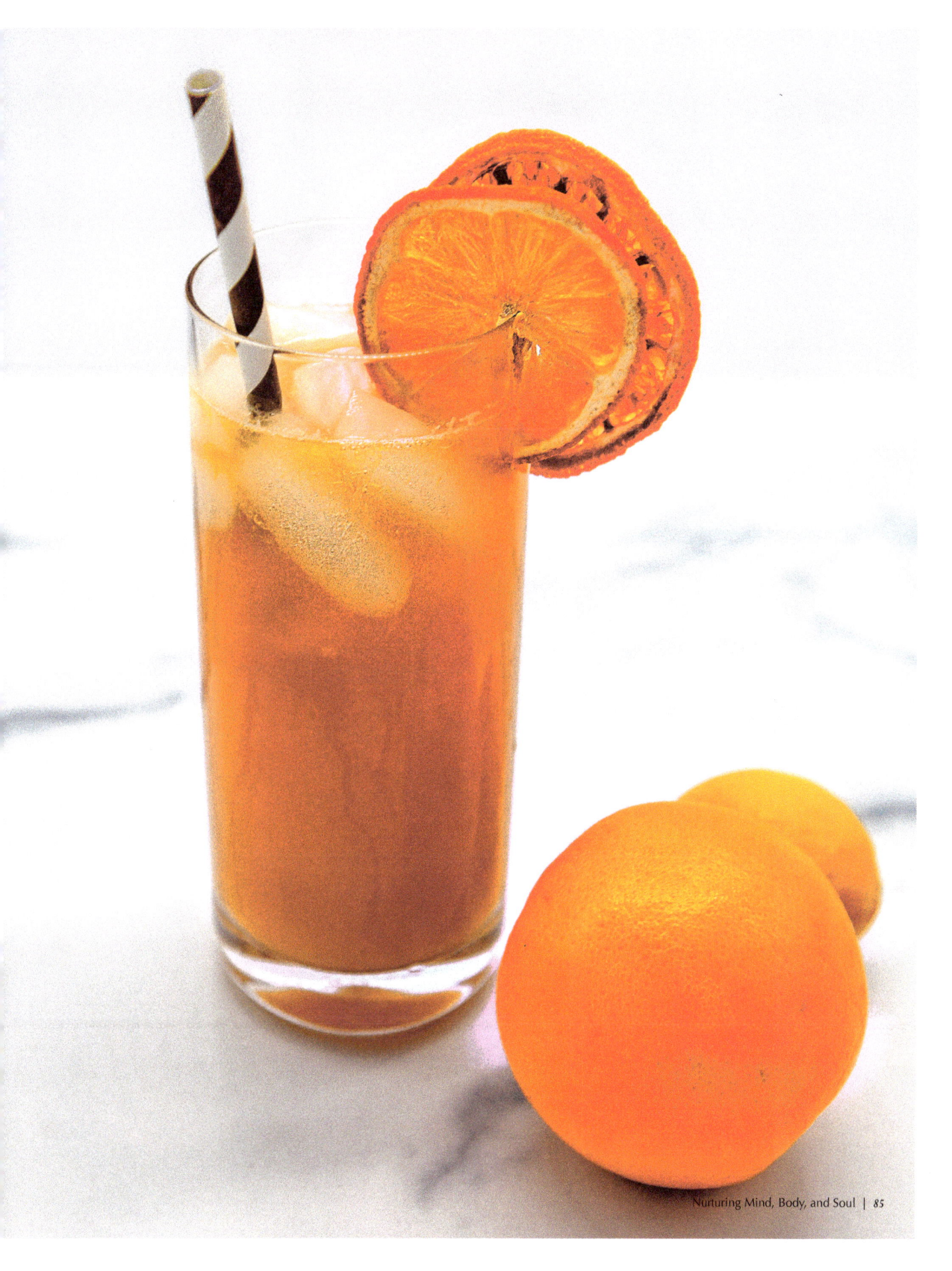

Yogurt Split

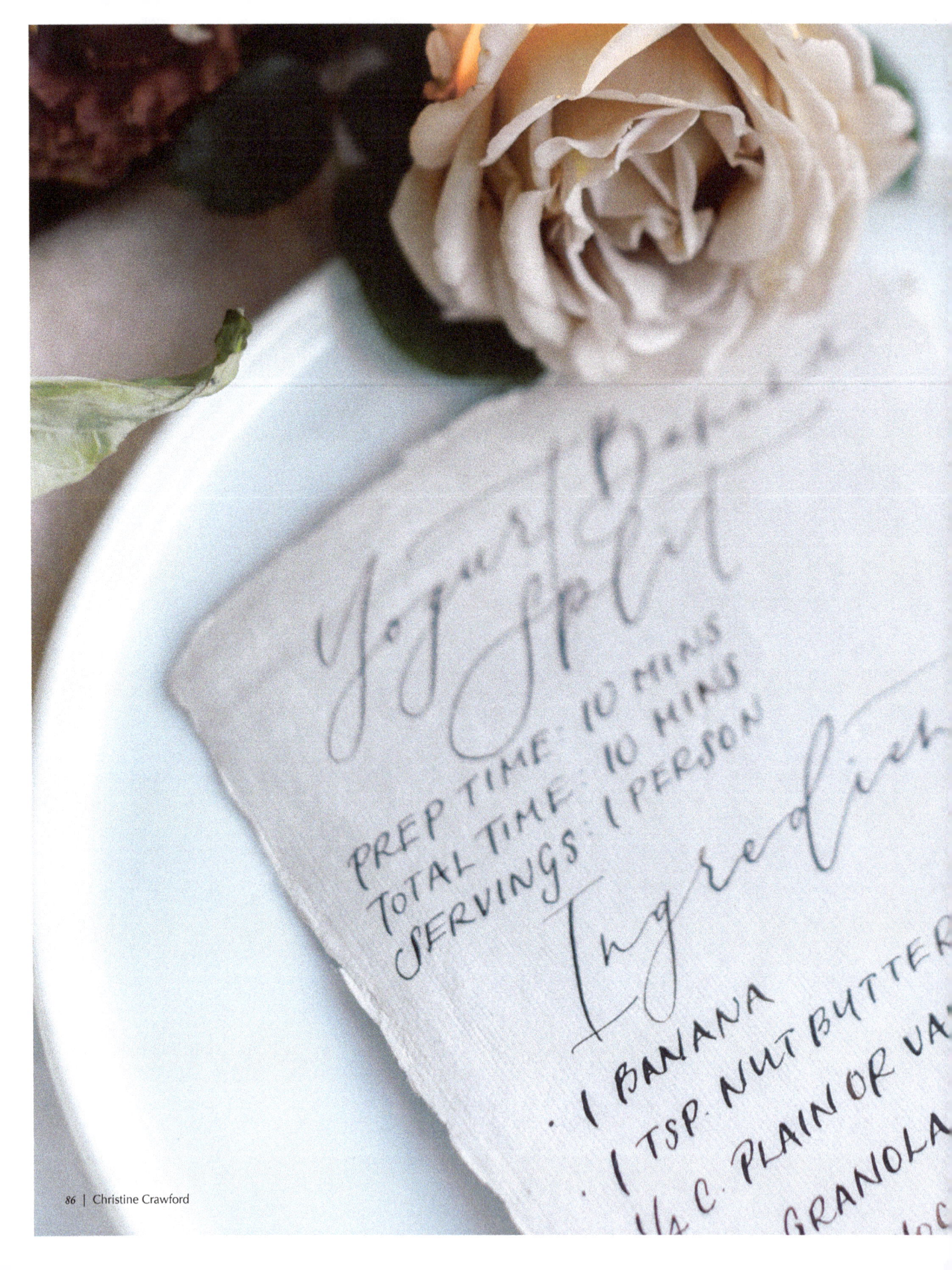

PREP TIME: 10 MINS
TOTAL TIME: 10 MINS
SERVINGS: 1 PERSON

Ingredients

- 1 BANANA
- 1 TSP. NUT BUTTER
- ½ C. PLAIN OR VA[NILLA]
- GRANOLA

YOGURT

Yogurt is a nutritious and beneficial food for many reasons. It is a fermented dairy product that introduces beneficial bacteria (such as Lactobacillus bulgaricus and Streptococcus thermophilus) to milks. These live bacteria, known as probiotics, populate the gut and help maintain a healthy gut flora balance. Probiotics can aid digestion, support the immune system, and even improve digestive conditions.

Yogurt is an excellent source of high-quality protein essential for tissue repair, muscle maintenance, growth, and development. Protein also helps keep us fuller for longer, making it an excellent addition to a balanced diet. It is rich in vitamins and minerals, including calcium, vitamin B12, riboflavin (vitamin B2), phosphorus, potassium, and magnesium. These nutrients are essential for various bodily functions, such as energy production, nerve function, and maintaining healthy cells.

Some studies suggest yogurt consumption may be associated with better weight management. The protein and probiotics in yogurt can help promote satiety and support a healthy metabolism. Regular yogurt consumption has been linked to a reduced risk of heart disease. The calcium, potassium, and probiotics in yogurt, along with its potential to lower LDL cholesterol, contribute to better heart health.

It's important to note that not all yogurts are created equal. When choosing yogurt, choose varieties with live and active cultures (look for "contains live and active cultures" on the label), and avoid those with added sugars and artificial ingredients. Greek yogurt and other plain, unsweetened varieties tend to be healthier choices.

YOGURT BANANA SPLIT

PREP TIME 10 minutes, TOTAL TIME 10 minutes
SERVINGS 1 Person

INGREDIENTS

- 1 banana
- 1 tbsp. nut butter
- 1/4 cup plain or vanilla yogurt
- 1/4 cup your favorite granola
- 1/4 bar chocolate
- 15 blueberries
- 1 strawberry

INSTRUCTIONS

1. Start by slicing a banana lengthwise.
2. Add a large scoop of nut butter, followed by a large scoop of yogurt, to the center.
3. Melt chocolate bar by microwaving for 30-second intervals, stirring between each, until melted.
4. Sprinkle with berries, granola, and chopped nuts. Use a spoon to drizzle with chocolate. Enjoy!

NOTES

TOPPING IDEAS: granola, chopped nuts, strawberries, raspberries, cherries, blueberries, dried cranberries, or shredded coconut.

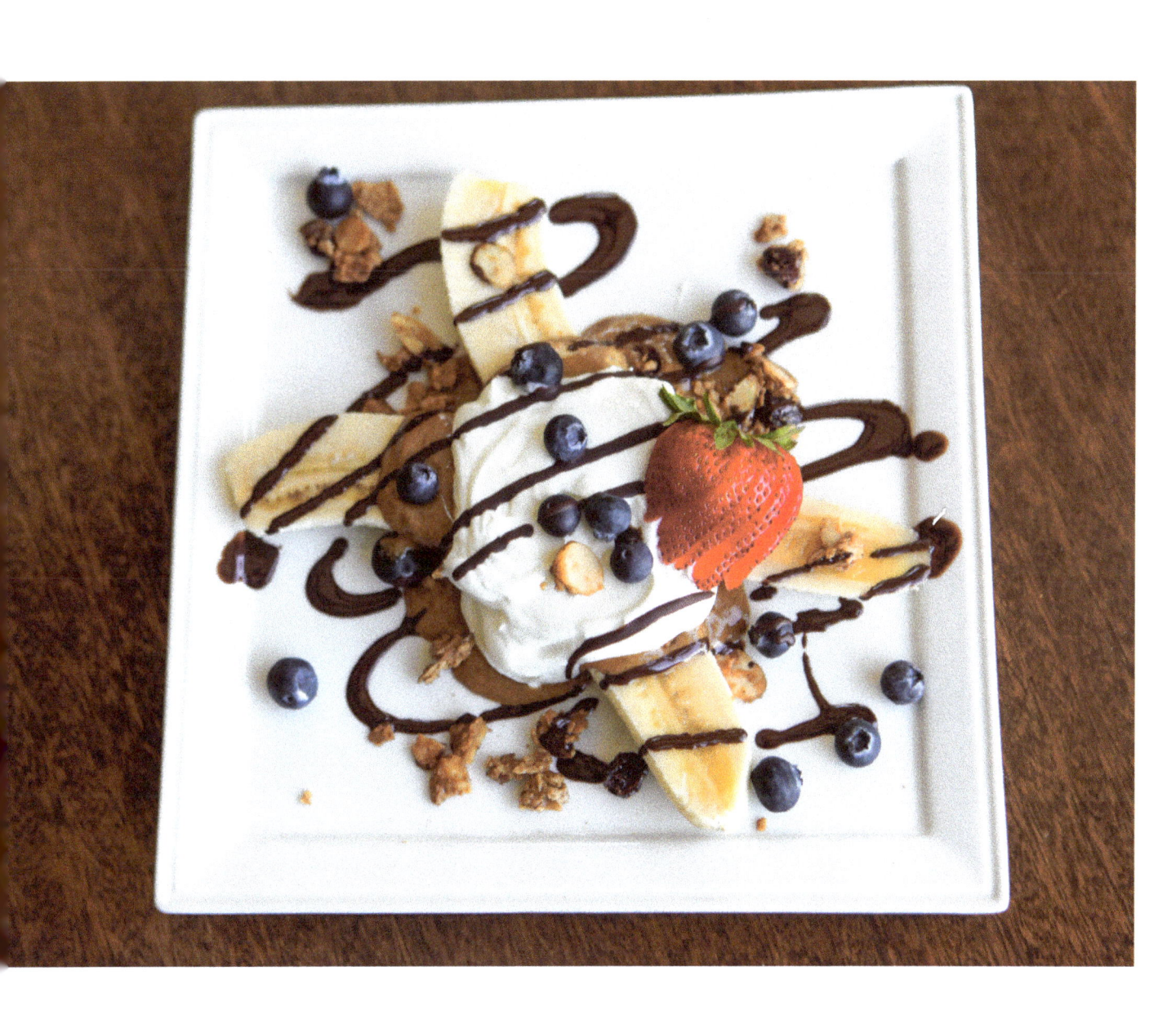

BLISTERED CHERRY TOMATOES AND YOGURT

This dish is adapted from Ottolenghi's charred tomato dish in his cookbook, Simple. The warm vibrant flavors of the roasted tomatoes are set off beautifully by the rich, cold, creaminess of the yogurt.

PREP TIME 10 minutes, TOTAL TIME 20 minutes
SERVINGS 4 People

INGREDIENTS

- 1 cup cherry tomatoes
- 1 tbsp. olive oil
- 1 tsp. dried oregano
- 1/2 tsp. dried thyme
- 1/2 tsp. paprika
- Salt and pepper to taste.
- 1 cup Greek yogurt
- Fresh basil leaves, for garnish

INSTRUCTIONS

1. Preheat your oven to a high broil setting.
2. In a mixing bowl, combine the cherry tomatoes, olive oil, dried oregano, dried thyme, paprika, salt, and pepper. Toss well to coat the tomatoes evenly with the Mediterranean spices.
3. Spread the coated cherry tomatoes on a baking sheet in a single layer.
4. Place the baking sheet with the tomatoes under the broiler for about 5-7 minutes or until the tomatoes start to blister and char, giving them a smoky flavor. Keep a close eye on them to prevent burning.
5. While the tomatoes are blistering, spoon the Greek yogurt onto a serving dish or individual bowls.
6. Once the cherry tomatoes are charred to your liking, remove them from the oven and let them cool slightly.
7. Spoon the blistered cherry tomatoes on top of the Greek yogurt.
8. Garnish with fresh basil leaves for added freshness and flavor.
9. Serve immediately and enjoy as a refreshing appetizer or light snack.
10. The Mediterranean spices like oregano, thyme, and paprika add a wonderful savory flavor to the blistered tomatoes, complementing the creamy Greek yogurt.

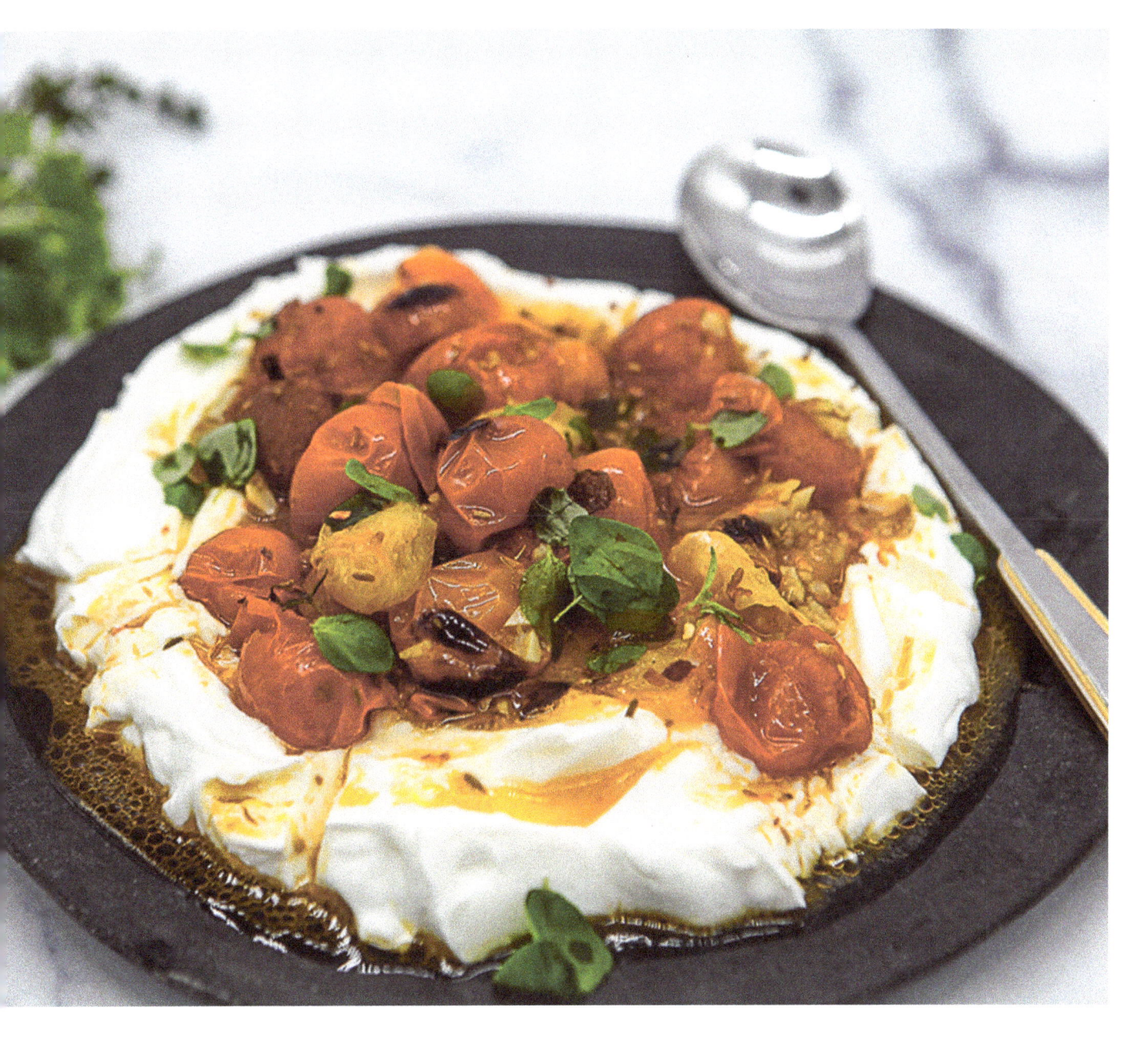

11. Feel free to adjust the spice quantities according to your taste preferences. You can also add other Mediterranean-inspired toppings like a drizzle of extra virgin olive oil or a sprinkle of crumbled feta cheese for added richness.

STRAWBERRY YOGURT POPSICLES

Did you know, adding apples, oranges and strawberries to your daily diet can help prevent cognitive decline?

PREP TIME 10 minutes, DOWNTIME 4-6 hours,
TOTAL TIME 4-6 hours 10 minutes, SERVINGS 8 popsicles

INGREDIENTS

- 2 cups fresh strawberries hulled and chopped.
- 1 cup plain Greek yogurt.
- 1/4 cup maple syrup (adjust to taste)
- 1/4 tsp. vanilla extract

INSTRUCTIONS

1. Place the chopped strawberries in a blender or food processor, and blend until smooth.
2. Combine the strawberry puree, Greek yogurt, maple syrup, and vanilla extract in a mixing bowl. Stir well.
3. Taste the mixture and adjust the sweetness if needed by adding more honey or maple syrup.
4. Pour the mixture into Popsicle molds.
5. Insert Popsicle sticks into each mold, ensuring they are upright and secure.
6. Place the molds in the freezer and let them freeze for at least 4-6 hours or until fully solidified.
7. Once the popsicles are frozen, remove them from the molds by briefly running them under warm water. This will help release the popsicles.

Enjoy your homemade strawberry yogurt popsicles immediately or store them in a sealed container or plastic bag in the freezer for later.

NOTES: You can also add chunks of fresh strawberries to the mixture, before pouring it into the molds for an added burst of fruity flavor and texture.

Nurturing Mind, Body, and Soul | 93

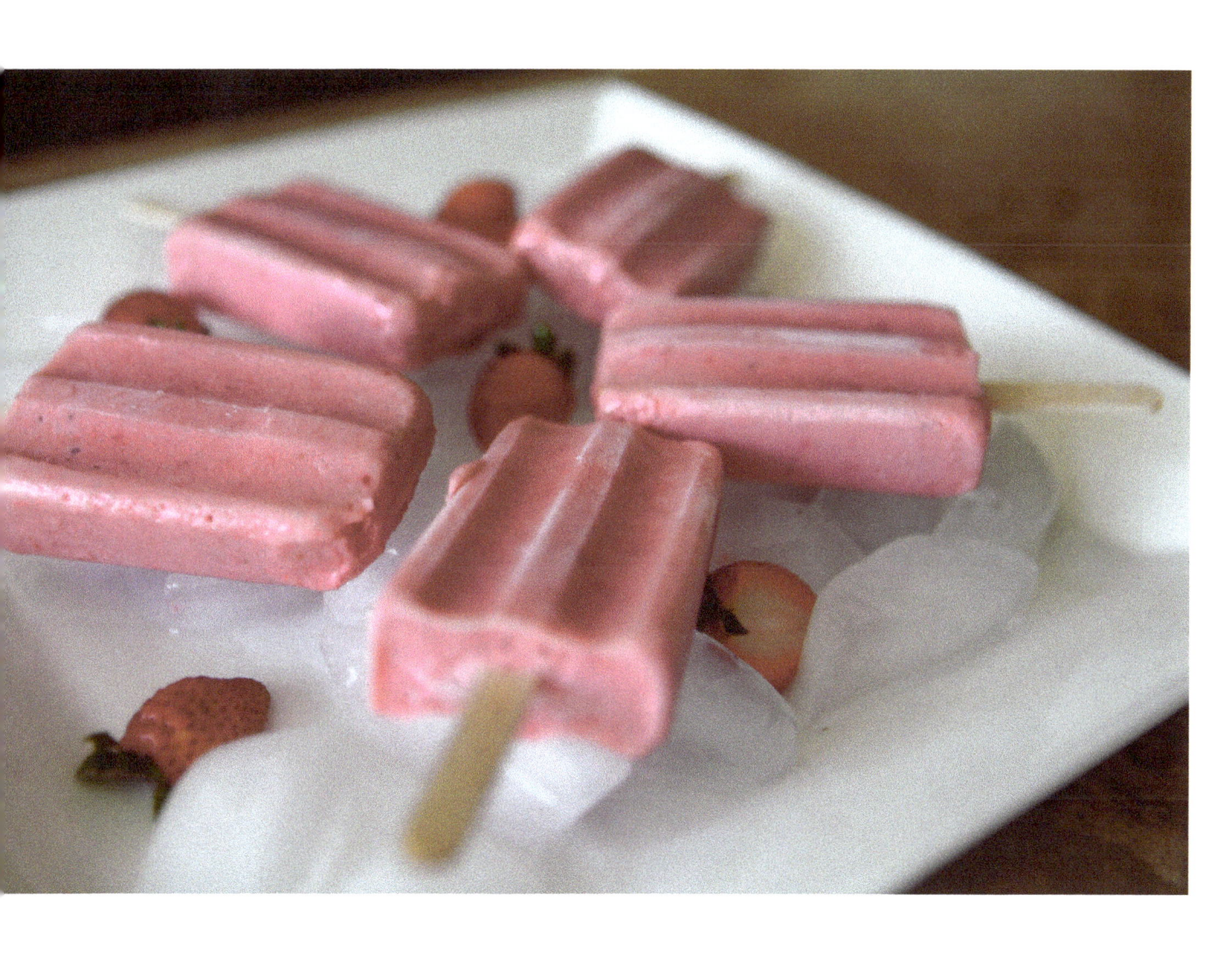

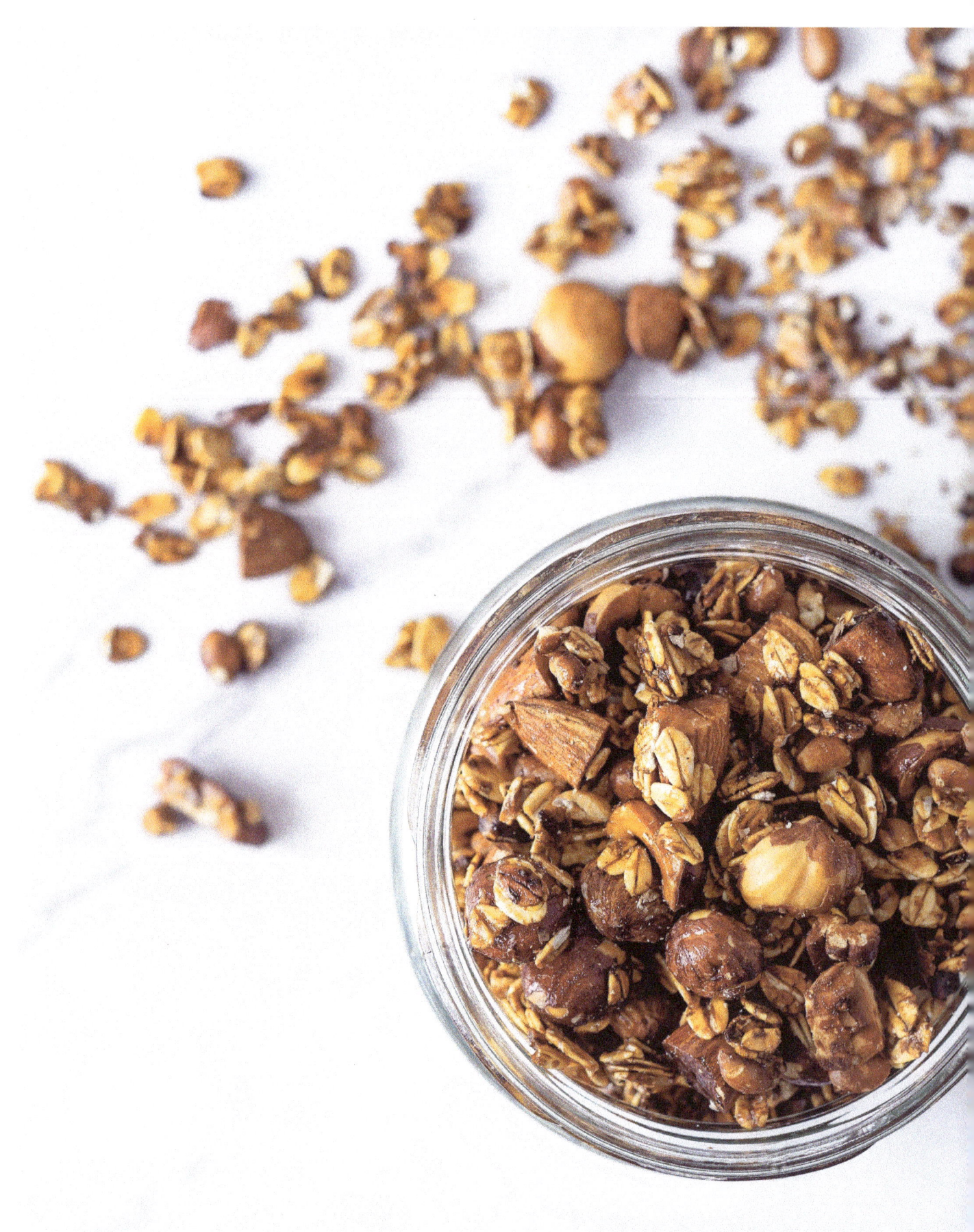

TOPPINGS & ADD-INS

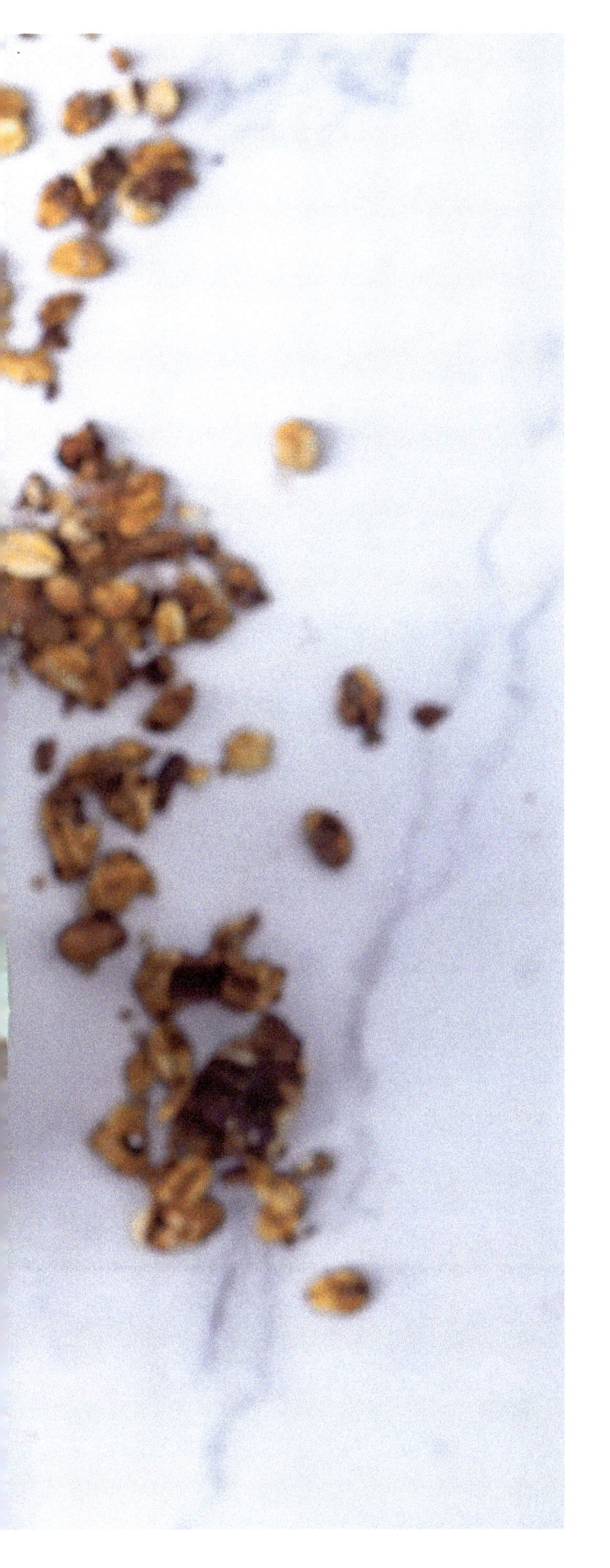

GRANOLA

Granola consists of rolled oats, nuts, seeds, dried fruits, sweeteners like maple syrup or palm sugar. When made and consumed mindfully, granola can offer numerous health benefits and a delightful taste experience.

It's important to be cautious about commercially available granola, which is often high in added sugars, unhealthy fats, and calories. If you're looking to reap the health benefits of granola, consider making it at home or carefully reading labels to find a product that aligns with your dietary preferences and needs.

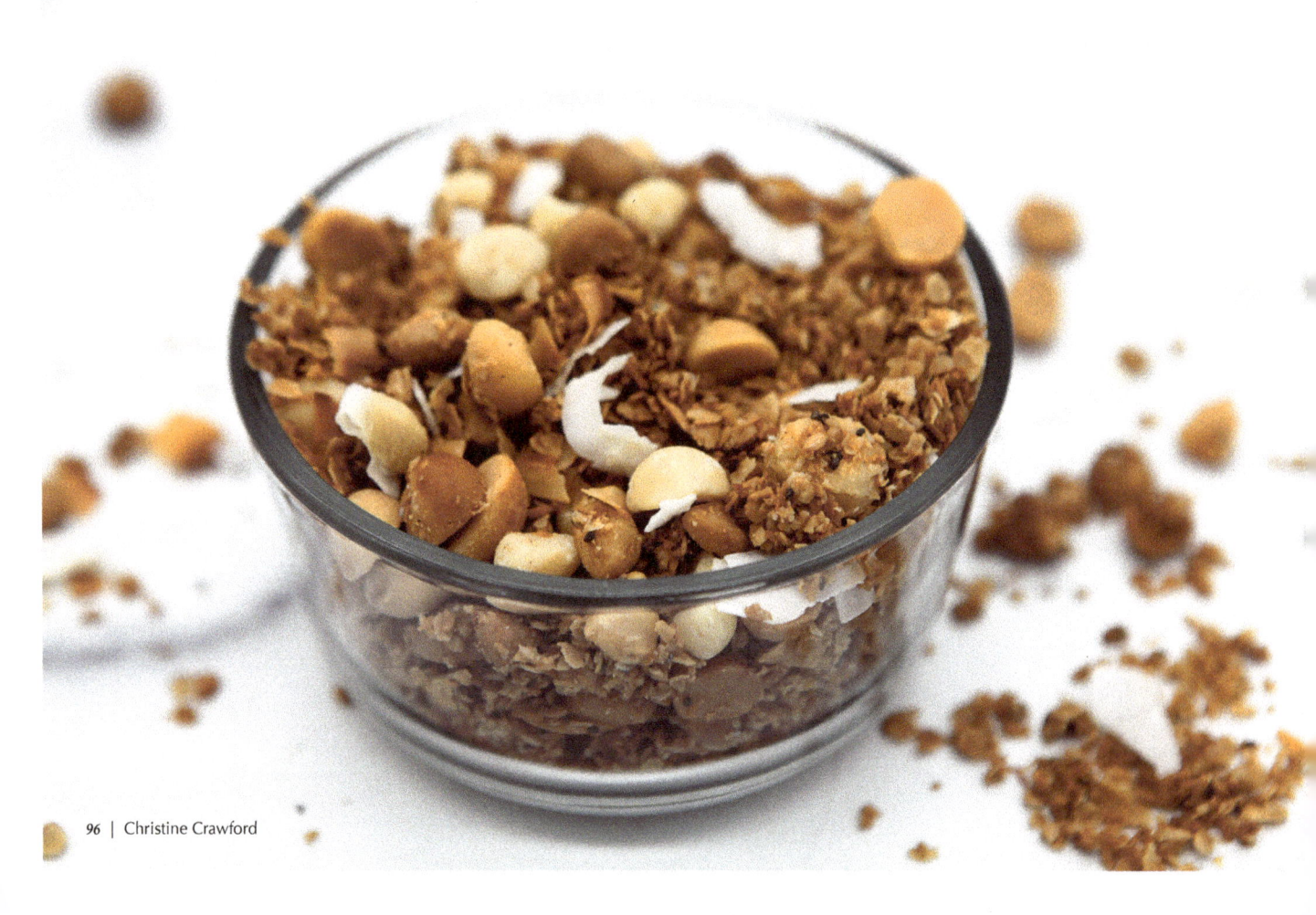

COCONUT MACADAMIA NUT GRANOLA

PREP TIME 5 minutes, COOK TIME 40 minutes
TOTAL TIME 45 minutes, SERVINGS 12

INGREDIENTS

- 2 1/2 cups old-fashioned oats use certified GF oats to keep GF
- 1 tbsp. flax seeds
- 1/2 tsp. sea salt
- 1/4 tsp. nutmeg
- 1 cup raw macadamia nuts
- 1 cup shredded coconut
- 1/3 cup extra virgin coconut oil melted
- 1 tbsp. vanilla extract
- 1/3 cup maple syrup

INSTRUCTIONS

1. Preheat oven to 300°F. Line a large baking sheet with parchment paper.
2. Combine oats, flax seeds, shaved coconut, and macadamia nuts in a large bowl. Whisk together the melted coconut oil, maple syrup, vanilla extract, and sea salt in a smaller bowl. Pour wet ingredients into dry ingredients and stir together until the dry ingredients are completely coated.
3. Spread the mixture evenly on the prepared baking sheet. Bake in the preheated oven for about 30-40 minutes. Stir the granola halfway through baking to ensure even browning and prevent the edges from burning. Remove from oven. If you like chunky granola, press down on it when it gets out of the oven (wear a glove if it's still hot).
4. Allow to cool and enjoy!
5. Store your coconut macadamia nut granola in an airtight container at room temperature. It should stay fresh for up to two weeks.

COMPOTES

Compotes are fruit-based sauces or preserves containing no added sugar or reduced sugar. Instead of relying on sugar to sweeten the compote, the natural sweetness of the fruits is enhanced and concentrated through the cooking process.

Here's how compotes work and why they can be sweet without added sugar:

Fruits contain natural sugars, such as fructose and glucose, which provide sweetness. When cooking down fruits in a compote, the natural sugars are released and become more concentrated, intensifying the sweetness of the compote.

Cooking a compote involves simmering fruits in a liquid (such as water or fruit juice) until they soften and break down. As the fruits cook, their natural sugars are released, and the liquid reduces to about half its volume, leading to a naturally sweet and thickened compote.

The fresh or frozen fruits used in compotes contain essential vitamins, minerals, and dietary fiber. These nutrients contribute to overall health and well-being. You can opt for low glycemic sweeteners like maple syrup or palm sugar if additional sweetness is desired. These alternatives have a lower impact on blood sugar levels than refined sugar.

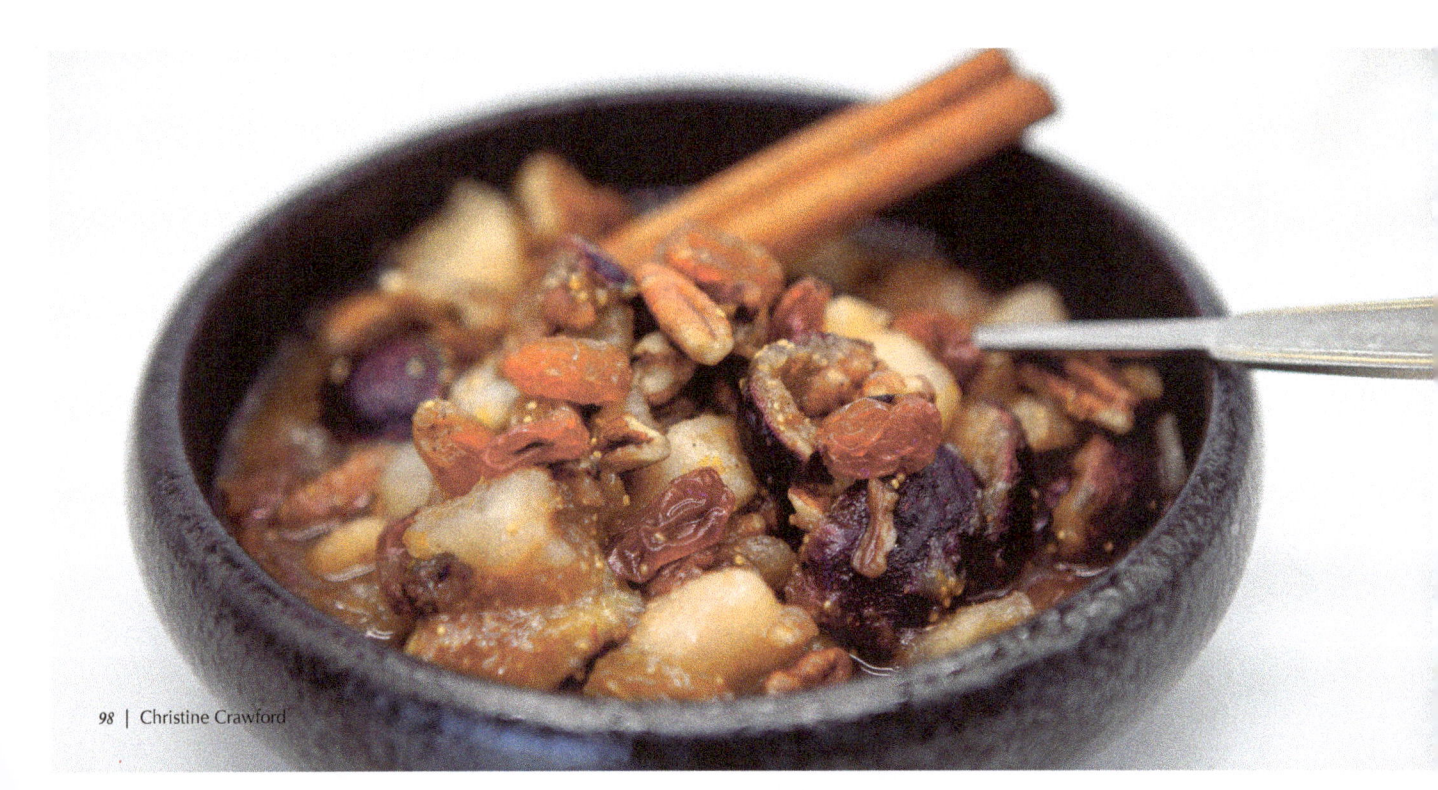

AUTUMN SPICED PEAR AND FIG COMPOTE, WITH RAISINS AND PECANS

PREP TIME 15 minutes, COOK TIME 20 minutes
TOTAL TIME 35 minutes, SERVINGS 10

INGREDIENTS

- 3 cups diced pears (Bosc or Anjou)
- 1 cup fresh figs, quartered
- 1/2 cup raisins, crimson or golden
- 1/2 cup apple juice
- 1/3 cup maple syrup (adjust to taste)
- 1 cinnamon stick
- 1/2 tsp. ground nutmeg
- A pinch of salt
- 1 tsp. vanilla extract (optional)
- 1/2 cup chopped toasted walnuts or pecans (optional for crunch)

INSTRUCTIONS

1. Preparation: Dice the pears and quarter the figs. Set aside.
2. Combine Ingredients: In a medium-sized saucepan, combine the diced pears, figs, raisins, apple juice, maple syrup, cinnamon stick, nutmeg, cloves, allspice, and a pinch of salt.
3. Simmer: Place the saucepan over medium heat. Once the mixture starts to bubble, reduce the heat to low and let it simmer for 20-30 minutes, stirring occasionally. The pears and figs should become tender, and the liquid should thicken into a syrupy consistency.
4. Final Touches: Once the fruits are tender, remove the saucepan from the heat and stir in the vanilla extract if using. If you like some crunch in your compote, you can stir in the toasted walnuts or pecans at this point.
5. Serve: Remove the cinnamon stick before serving. This compote is excellent both warm and at room temperature. It pairs beautifully with yogurt, oatmeal, toast, pancakes, or even roasted meats.
6. Storage: Store any leftovers in an airtight container in the refrigerator for up to a week. Warm it up slightly before serving if desired.

NOTES

This recipe is flexible, and you can easily adjust the spices and sweetness to your liking. Enjoy your autumn treat!

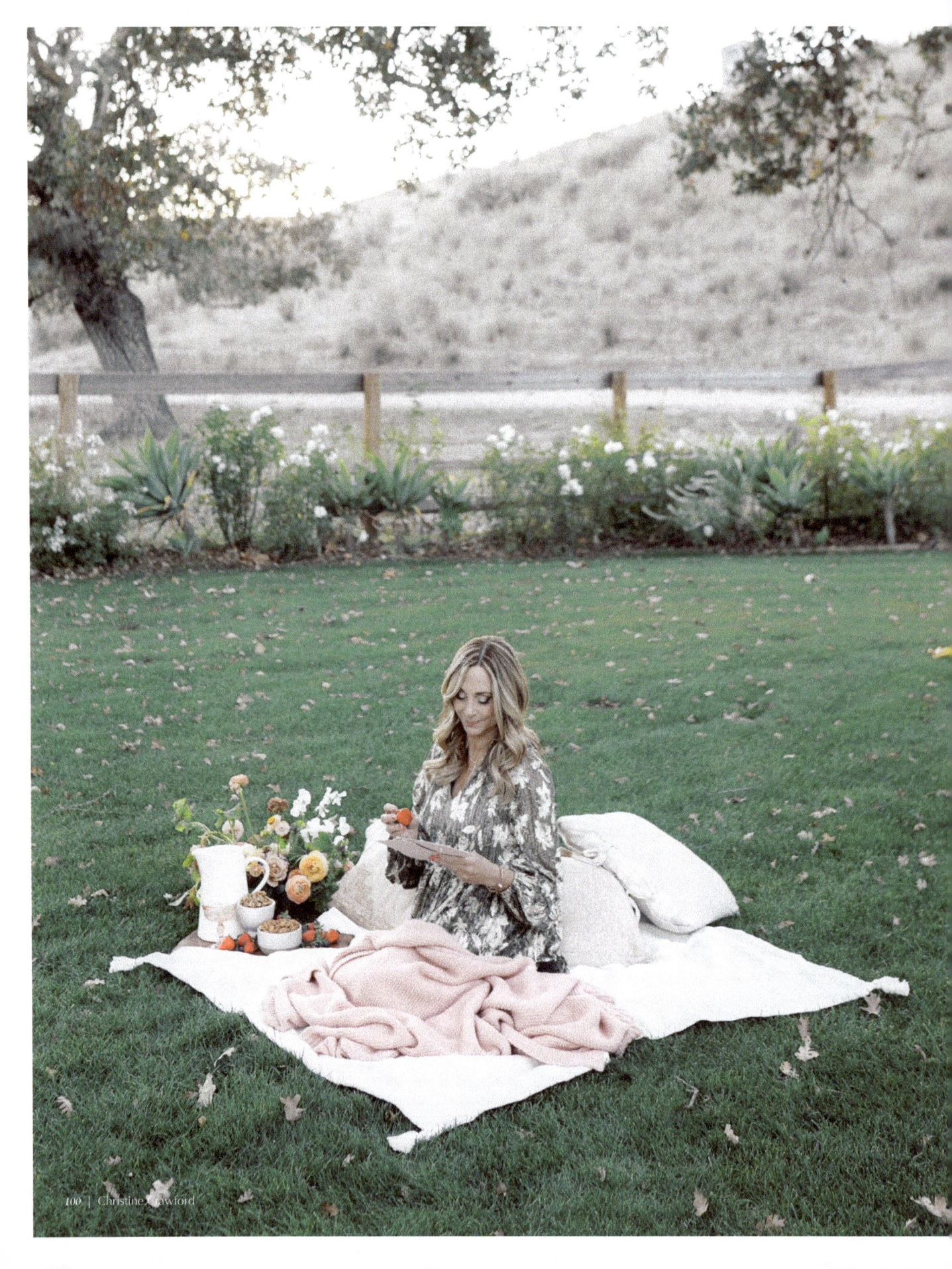

Printed in the USA
CPSIA information can be obtained
at www.ICGtesting.com
CBHW041710070824
12782CB00039B/696

9 798989 359004